SOCIAL INEQUALITY AND PUBLIC HEALTH

Edited by Salvatore J. Babones

This edition published in Great Britain in 2009 by

The Policy Press
University of Bristol
Fourth Floor
Beacon House
Queen's Road
Bristol BS8 1QU
UK

Tel +44 (0)117 331 4054
Fax +44 (0)117 331 4093
e-mail tpp-info@bristol.ac.uk
www.policypress.org.uk

North American office:
The Policy Press
c/o International Specialized Books Services (ISBS)
920 NE 58th Avenue, Suite 300
Portland, OR 97213-3786, USA
Tel +1 503 287 3093
Fax +1 503 280 8832
e-mail info@isbs.com

British Library Cataloguing in Publication Data
A catalogue record for this book is available from the British Library.

Library of Congress Cataloging-in-Publication Data
A catalog record for this book has been requested.

ISBN 978 1 84742 320 7 paperback
ISBN 978 1 84742 321 4 hardcover

The right of Salvatore J. Babones to be identified as editor of this work has been asserted
by him in accordance with the 1988 Copyright, Designs and Patents Act.

Cover design by Qube Design Associates, Bristol
Front cover: image kindly supplied by www.alamy.com
Printed and bound in Great Britain by Hobbs the Printers, Southampton

Contents

List of figures, tables, maps and boxes

Figures

Tables

Maps

Box

Preface

This volume explores the relationship between social inequality and public health. Health in every society is stratified by income, race and class. Rich people enjoy better health than poor people; members of the majority enjoy better health than members of disadvantaged minorities; professionals enjoy better health than workers. It had long been assumed that these social gradients in health resulted from differential access to healthcare or systematically different health behaviours between groups: lower-ranked groups could not get medical care, or smoked more or simply did not trust doctors. Mounting evidence, however, suggests that more is at work. Social scientists and public health researchers are becoming increasingly convinced that the social context in which an individual lives has a powerful direct effect on health, independent of health resources and behaviours. Moreover, entire societies seem to have better health outcomes than others; on this count, the US, the richest country the world has ever known, scores particularly badly. We are only beginning to understand the links between societal inequality and individual health; this volume represents a survey of research on the subject, written by scholars who are actively engaged in pushing forward the state of the art.

The individual chapters collected here emerged out of conversations held at the 2006 Pitt International Conference on Inequality, Health and Society. The organisers – Siddharth Chandra, John Marx, Ravi Sharma, Ken Thompson and myself – brought together leading social science and public health scholars from around the world to discuss ways to improve our understanding of how societal inequality affects broad population health. The chapters represented in this volume emphatically are not reprints of papers presented at the conference. On the contrary, most of the chapters were written expressly for this volume. In fact, several of the contributors did not even attend the conference, but were nonetheless eager to participate in this book project. One reason is that many of us researching the relationship between social inequality and public health see a pressing need to educate health and health policy professionals – not just academics – about the importance of societal context in influencing individual health outcomes. The chapters in this volume, accordingly, take quite sophisticated academic propositions, strip them of their customary statistical argumentation and present them in words and figures in a language that non-specialists can understand. The result is a volume that is rigorous without being arcane.

Editing this book has been both an honour and a pleasure. I have had the opportunity to work closely with many of the best minds at work today on problems of population health. A casual glance at the contributor list will confirm just how lucky I have been. I am indebted to them not only for their contributions to this volume, but much more for their contributions to my own intellectual development. Many thanks are also owed to the students who worked with me both in organising the conference and in putting together this volume.

In alphabetical order, they are Kevin Doran, Kandi Felmet, Paula Ilochi, Aimee Moore, Leah Taylor and Kelly Thomas. They were indispensable. Staff members of the University of Pittsburgh's Department of Sociology, University Center for International Studies and Graduate School of Public Health all contributed as well. Funding for the project that ultimately resulted in this volume was provided by the University of Pittsburgh's Global Studies Program, Office of the Provost, Graduate School of Public Health, European Union Center for Excellence/ European Studies Center and Graduate School of Public and International Affairs. Through many conversations over the course of this project, Ravi Sharma and Siddharth Chandra made major contributions to my thinking on the public health of social inequality.

I owe a special debt of gratitude to four people who were instrumental in bringing this project to fruition: Michael Ames, Jim Dunn, Mary Shaw and the Director of The Policy Press, Alison Shaw.

Last and unforgettably, I owe a heartfelt thank you to John Marx and Ken Thompson for all their support over the past five years. This project would never have been conceived or executed without them. I am glad they pushed me into it. While it is tempting to claim that any remaining deficiencies in this work are theirs, I am sure that they are, in fact, mine. I am also quite sure they know that even better than I do.

Salvatore J. Babones
Department of Sociology and Social Policy
The University of Sydney, Australia
October 2008

Notes on contributors

Jean Adams is a Lecturer in Public Health in the Institute of Health and Society at Newcastle University, UK. Her research focuses on socioeconomic inequalities in health behaviours and health. She is currently working on projects studying food advertising; and socioeconomic inequalities in the provision of cancer care.

Ronald J. Angel is Professor of Sociology at the University of Texas at Austin, USA. His work focuses on the social welfare state and the role of non-governmental organizations (NGOs) in service delivery. His most recent book is *Poor Families in America's Health Care Crisis* (with Laura Lein and Jane Henrici) (Cambridge University Press, 2006).

Salvatore J. Babones is a Lecturer in the Department of Sociology and Social Policy at The University of Sydney, Australia. His research centres on the study of income inequality, its causes, and its effects. His book *The International Structure of Income: Its Implications for Economic Growth* has just been published by VDM Press (2008).

Debbie Barrington is Assistant Professor of Epidemiology at Columbia University's Mailman School of Public Health, USA. Her primary research interests include the social epidemiology of racial/ethnic disparities in perinatal outcomes, and the effects of nativity status and intergenerational factors on the health of African-Americans.

Stephen Bezruchka, an emergency physician, is Senior Lecturer in the Departments of Global Health and Health Services, School of Public Health and Community Medicine, University of Washington, Seattle, USA. His work centres on disseminating concepts of population health. He received the School's 2002 Outstanding Teacher Award and the 2008 Faculty Community Service Award.

Martin Bobak is Professor of Epidemiology in Division of Population Health at University College London, UK. His research interests focus on health in the former communist countries of Central and Eastern Europe, particularly the interplay between socioeconomic and psychosocial factors and health behaviours.

Eric Brunner is a Reader in the Department of Epidemiology and Public Health at University College London, UK. He is a Principal Investigator on the Whitehall II Study of social inequalities in health and Co-director of the Health and Society: Social Epidemiology Masters course.

Siddharth Chandra is Associate Professor of Economics in the Graduate School of Public and International Affairs at the University of Pittsburgh, USA. His research combines concepts from economics and psychology to analyse problems related to addiction and identity. His recent publications have appeared in the journals *Drug and Alcohol Dependence, Journal of Research in Personality*, and *Experimental and Clinical Psychopharmacology*.

James R. Dunn holds a Chair in Applied Public Health from the Canadian Institutes of Health Research and the Public Health Agency of Canada. He is a Research Scientist at the Centre for Research on Inner City Health at St Michael's Hospital, Toronto, and an Associate Professor in the Departments of Geography & Planning and Public Health Sciences at the University of Toronto.

Annie Feighery is a PhD candidate and policy fellow in International Educational Development at Teachers College, Columbia University, USA. She researches urban poverty and health, humanitarian responses to climate change, and international development policy.

Tamara Dubowitz is an Associate Policy Researcher at the RAND Corporation, USA. Her research focuses on the policy ramifications of social determinants of health. Her major interests include examination of neighbourhood effects (for example the built physical and social environment) on obesity and diet-related disease.

Maryann Z. Fiebach is a Master of Public Health candidate at the Columbia University Mailman School of Public Health, USA, as part of the Urbanism and the Built Environment track of the Department of Sociomedical Sciences. Her MPH thesis examines housing quality and self-reported health status in New York City.

Clyde Hertzman is the President of the Canadian Council on Early Child Development, Director of the Human Early Learning Partnership and Professor in the School of Population and Public Health at the University of British Columbia. He is a Fellow of the Canadian Institute for Advanced Research, a Canada Research Chair in Population Health and Human Development, and a Fellow of the Royal Society of Canada.

Peter Heywood is the Director of Public Health for Middlesbrough Primary Care Trust and Middlesbrough Council, UK. He was previously Clinical Lecturer in Public Health at Newcastle University. His research and evaluation work focuses on the prevention and early management of cardiovascular disease and diabetes in disadvantaged communities.

Kristen Kurland is a Teaching Professor at Carnegie Mellon University's Heinz College and School of Architecture, Pittsburgh, USA. Her research focuses on interdisciplinary collaborations in health and the built environment, and advanced spatial analysis using geographic information systems. She is the co-author of a series of GIS workbooks for ESRI Press.

Emily Karpel Kurtz is the Assistant Director, Special Projects at the Ridgewood Bushwick Senior Citizens Council, Inc in Brooklyn, New York, USA. She served as a research assistant to Professors Northridge and Sclar in 2003, during which time she conducted preliminary research for the chapter published here.

Paul Nelson is Associate Professor in the Graduate School of Public and International Affairs, University of Pittsburgh, USA, where he directs the International Development programme. He teaches and conducts research on human rights, development policy, NGOs, and religion and development. He is the author, with Ellen Dorsey, of *New Rights Advocacy* (Georgetown University Press, 2008).

Mary E. Northridge is Professor of Clinical Sociomedical Sciences at the Columbia University Mailman School of Public Health, USA. She holds a joint appointment in the College of Dental Medicine, and is a faculty member in the Urban Planning Program, where she teaches a cross-listed course titled 'Interdisciplinary Planning for Health'.

Theresa L. Osypuk is an Assistant Professor at Northeastern University Bouvé College of Health Sciences, USA. She is a social epidemiologist researching how place and residential segregation matter for racial/ethnic health disparities. Her research has been published recently in *American Journal of Epidemiology*, *Health Affairs*, and *Urban Affairs Review*.

Javier Pereira Bruno is Professor and Chair of the Social Science Department at the Universidad Católica del Uruguay in Montevideo, Uruguay. His research examines the nature of non-governmental public action, particularly in the field of children and adolescent policy. He has held Fulbright, National Science Foundation and Andrew Mellon Fellowships.

Nancy A. Ross is an Associate Professor in the Department of Geography at McGill University in Montreal, Canada. She also holds appointments with the Department of Epidemiology, Biostatistics and Occupational Health at McGill University and Statistics Canada. Her research is concerned with social and economic determinants of health in urban environments.

Elliott D. Sclar is Professor of Urban Planning and International Affairs at the Columbia University Graduate School of Architecture, Planning and Preservation and School of International and Public Affairs, USA.

Arjumand Siddiqi is Assistant Professor at the University of the Gillings School of Global Public Health at the University of North Carolina, Chapel Hill, and Faculty Fellow of the Carolina Population Center, USA. She is interested in the role of social investment strategies in shaping inequities in population health and human development.

Martin White is Professor of Public Health in the Institute of Health & Society at Newcastle University, UK, and Director of the UKCRC-funded Centre for Translational Research in Public Health. His research focuses on the development and evaluation of public health interventions, and understanding and tackling inequalities in health.

Richard Wilkinson trained in economic history and epidemiology. He worked briefly in the British National Health Service before taking up research on health inequalities and the social determinants of health. He is Emeritus Professor (Social Epidemiology) at the University of Nottingham, and Honorary Professor at University College London and at the University of York, UK.

ONE

Introduction

Salvatore J. Babones

In 1916, epidemiologist Hibbert Winslow Hill published an influential volume on *The new public health* of his day, which was increasingly focused on the individual-level biological determinants of health. In Hill's synopsis, 'the old public health was concerned with the environment; the new is concerned with the individual' (Hill, 1916, p 8). The individual-level orientation of this 'new public health' was explicitly formulated in reaction to the 'old public health' of the 19th century, in which founding epidemiologists like John Snow had uncovered the environmental origins of major diseases like cholera. As the 20th century dawned, advances in cell biology were leading to a shift of the centre of gravity of epidemiology out of the field and into the laboratory. Disease came to be seen as something that affected a person, not a population. So far as the new public health of the early 20th century was concerned, populations were nothing more than aggregations of individuals. In this mode of thought, improving public health came down to improving the individual health of as many people as possible.

The 'new public health' of the early 21st century has come full circle. The past two decades have witnessed the emergence of a 'new' new public health focused on how social, economic and political factors affect the level and distribution of individual health. The emergence of this 21st-century new public health has to some extent been inspired by the success of 20th-century public health in battling disease within the individual. Today, the most serious public health challenges facing the populations of the high-income countries of Europe, North America and North East Asia are mainly preventable, or at least treatable, diseases. As a result, environmental factors (broadly construed) are now more important for understanding differences in the health of individuals than ever before. The most important of these environmental factors are related to the social structures in which people are embedded. In high-income countries, where most people enjoy relatively good access to shelter, warmth, adequate nutrition, sanitation, clean drinking water and the like, social inequalities have become a major focus of public health research.

The impact of social inequalities on the level and distribution of population health is not, however, felt only in high-income countries. In poor countries as well, household income and assets are strongly correlated with a myriad of health outcomes, as demonstrated by the US AID Demographic and Health Surveys. If these effects are more apparent in high-income countries than in less-developed countries, it is only because less-developed countries suffer a high burden of preventable and treatable diseases as well. The impact of social inequality is ubiquitous, both within and across societies.

Today's new public health seeks to understand how the social environment affects health, with the ultimate goal of improving health by improving the social environments in which people live. This has led to a direct confrontation with the main public health research tradition of the 20th century: methodological individualism. That public health outcomes are socially patterned is not in dispute. What is very hotly contested, however, is the nature of the pathways that connect these social patterns to individual health. Four such pathways are examined in this volume, ranging from the well accepted to the highly controversial: health behaviour, group disadvantage, individual psychosocial factors and societal psychosocial factors. The first two pathways are now well accepted. The third is becoming clearer, in large part as a result of the definitive work of Michael Marmot and his colleagues with the Whitehall II Study of British civil servants. The last is the subject of fierce debate: advocated most prominently by Richard Wilkinson, it posits that there may be entire societies that are less healthy to live in than others because of the character of their social structures. If it is ultimately proved correct, it would turn Hill's individualistic 'new public health' of the early 20th century completely on its head.

The present volume is organised around these four pathways identified in the new public health of the 21st century as mechanisms through which social inequality affects public health. They are considered in four sections arranged in order from least to most controversial. The chapters in the first section, 'Pathway 1: Differences in individual health behaviours', examine how individual choices can be shaped by the alternatives offered in the environments in which people live. The chapters in the second section, 'Pathway 2: Group advantage and disadvantage', aggregate environments like those examined in Pathway 1 into larger syndromes affecting broad groups in society. The chapters in the third section, 'Pathway 3: Psychosocial factors in individual health', leap to an analytical level where the proximate (not just ultimate) cause of individual health is hypothesised to operate at the social level. The chapters in the fourth section, 'Pathway 4: Healthy and unhealthy societies', debate the more expansive hypothesis that entire societies can possess more or less healthy social structures. A concluding section addresses 'Public understanding of the new public health'.

The first major pathway through which larger social inequalities can affect public health is through the very direct mechanism of their effects on individual health behaviour. In Chapter Two, Jean Adams shows how social inequalities affect the way people think about the future, and through this affect their decisions to engage in health-destroying behaviours like smoking or avoiding health check-ups. In high-inequality societies, those on the lowest rungs of the socioeconomic ladder may not feel much incentive to plan for the long term, and as a result end up living in worse health when they get older. This can act as a drag on the public's health more broadly. This effect of the overall social environment on health is made more concrete by Tamara Dubowitz and colleagues in Chapter Three, who show how poverty in a high-inequality society (the US) is spatially associated with factors that make healthy living more difficult: a lack of quality food outlets and green spaces. The result is that people of low socioeconomic status must work harder to achieve the same level of health as people of high socioeconomic status. Not surprisingly, they end up, on average, living in poorer health. Mary E. Northridge and colleagues, writing in Chapter Four, pick up this thread, arguing for better community planning to promote healthy behaviours on a wide scale in both developed and developing countries.

The second major pathway through which social inequality affects public health is through the cumulative effects of advantage and disadvantage on broad population groups. Martin White and colleagues lay out a theoretical model for this in Chapter Five, showing how in the presence of social inequalities even interventions designed to improve health can widen health disparities between groups. For example, requiring cancer screening at medical examinations might be a laudable public health intervention, but in a society where not everyone is covered by health insurance, it tends to widen health disparities even as it improves overall health. In Chapter Six, Debbie Barrington takes up perhaps the most insidious case of group health disparities in the developed world, the gap between black and white people in the US. She traces the intergenerational aspects of the health deficit suffered by African Americans, likening the African American population to a canary in the coalmine: their multiply-disadvantaged status concentrates the health-depressing effects of social inequality. Javier Pereira Bruno and Ronald Angel describe health inequalities of a similar scale in Chapter Seven, although based on income rather than explicitly race, in Chile and Uruguay. In these countries, non-governmental organisations seeking to improve the health of the poor have historically had to work in direct opposition to the political power of repressive regimes. Today, both these countries are democratic, but healthcare for the poor still depends more on civil society than on governments.

The fact that material social inequalities based on income, racial discrimination, access to healthcare and the like are reflected in both individual and group health outcomes is now well accepted. More provocative is the idea that the social environment itself can affect individual health, the third major pathway examined in this book. In Chapter Eight, Eric Brunner uses data from the Whitehall II Study to show how low levels of control over one's own daily work can lead to high levels of stress that have both indirect and direct effects on health. The indirect effects, through behaviours such as smoking, are covered in Pathway 1. But Brunner goes further to argue that the workplace environment directly affects human biology. This is the crux of Pathway 3. In Chapter Nine, Siddharth Chandra traces out the ramifications of a very different effect of social inequality: its impact on identity formation. He argues that social inequalities directly affect how people perceive their world and themselves, and that this ultimately can have very broad implications for peace and governance in modern multi-group societies: a combination of Pathways 2 and 3. Arjumand Siddiqi and colleagues, writing in Chapter Ten, demonstrate how the population-wide effect of proximate psychosocial factors on public health can be truly enormous. They argue that the social shocks associated with the transition to capitalism in the 1990s in Eastern Europe are responsible for a massive increase in cardiovascular disease among working-age men.

The fourth – and most daring – hypothesised pathway through which social inequality can affect public health is through its connection with the character of society as a whole. The hypothesis, in a nutshell, is that less equal societies are simply less healthy social environments in which to live out one's life. Richard Wilkinson, the best-known proponent of this view, lays out the evidence to support this proposition in Chapter Eleven. He argues that inequality breeds status anxiety, individualism and consumerism, and that these forces threaten not only the individual health of all members of society but also the quality of the collective environment in which individuals must live. James R. Dunn and Nancy A. Ross use data on income inequality in US and Canadian cities to argue in Chapter Twelve that the relationship between social inequality and broad population health is itself contingent on the character of the societies in which people live: low-inequality countries (like Canada) incubate a culture of social solidarity, which potentially insulates individuals from the negative health effects of social inequality. They thus argue that it is possible to create a virtuous cycle in which policies that improve everyone's health (like universal healthcare) also promote social solidarity, which not only further improves everyone's health but also creates support for the policies that kicked off the cycle. In my own chapter, Chapter Thirteen, I come to a similar conclusion, arguing that reducing the harshness of today's rationalised workplaces would both improve health and reduce inequality at the same time.

Arguing the science behind the new public health is one thing; getting policy makers and the public to listen is quite another. Most of the countries of the world today are either democracies or, through the influence of the major intergovernmental organisations, encouraged to pursue policies promoted by the leading democracies. Accordingly, the final section of this book brings together three perspectives on how to promote public acceptance of the policy implications of the new public health. In Chapter Fourteen, Stephen Bezruchka calls the new public health 'a scientific revolution in progress' that is 'resisted by both scientists and the general population'. He calls for a broad-based education effort, focused not just on the schools but also on community activism, the internet and the press. Paul Nelson shows in Chapter Fifteen how emerging global human rights norms are being successfully used by civil society groups to drive pro-health policies in both developing and donor countries. This is occurring despite the fact that developed donor countries show little inclination to work towards meeting the health goals that they themselves set in international treaties. Civil society actors in poor countries in particular are relying on human rights narratives, not official treaty commitments, to prod their states into action on health. In my conclusion, Chapter Sixteen, I argue that the stakes of inaction on policies to promote public health are nothing less than the health of the world's democracies themselves.

Academic fashions do not so much come in cycles as spirals: each new innovation takes the last as its starting point. Nothing useful is ever discarded. The 'old' new public health of laboratory epidemiology has brought about a staggering expansion in our understanding of public health and is now the indispensable core of the discipline. Our increasing appreciation for the extent to which public health is shaped by social reality (and harmed by social inequality) in no way diminishes the importance of understanding the biological realities of public health. It does, however, open up new vistas that are difficult to survey from the laboratory bench. Even if social inequalities are, on average, responsible for just a one-year reduction in life expectancy, the disease burden due to social inequality would be equivalent to over 100 million lost life years annually worldwide. Taken together, the evidence presented in this volume collectively suggests that the benchmark of a one-year loss in life expectancy is conservative. Yet even this conservative benchmark would make social inequality a greater health challenge than cancer or AIDS. This is not an alarmist exaggeration; the total burden through all channels is almost certainly much higher. If this seems unrealistic, it is because social inequality is a diffuse public health challenge like obesity or air pollution: the fact that the impacts are spread widely across the population does not make them any less real.

When it comes to social inequality, however, there is a tragic irony in the fact that the powerful, privileged people who are best positioned to stem the epidemic are exactly the people who are least likely to suffer its consequences. After a century of general decline, social inequalities of all kinds are now on the rise in nearly every country of the world. The world's business, civic and even medical leaders all stand to benefit directly and very personally from rising inequality. Convincing them that lower inequality is in the public interest, or forcing them to accept inequality reductions via the ballot box, will surely be a difficult task. It is nonetheless one well worth pursuing.

References

Hill, H. W. (1916) *The new public health*, New York: Macmillan.

Pathway1
Differences in individual health behaviours

The role of time preference and perspective in socioeconomic inequalities in health-related behaviours

Jean Adams

Introduction

Pervasive socioeconomic inequalities in health and disease have been consistently reported within and between populations (Mackenbach et al, 1997; Acheson, 1998). While epidemiologists are adept at describing these relationships, evidence for interventions that can achieve whole-scale reduction of socioeconomic inequalities in health remains scarce (Arblaster et al, 1996; Gunning-Schepers and Gepkens, 1996; Alvarez-Dardet and Ashton, 2005). Socioeconomic differences in behaviours that influence health, such as smoking, diet and uptake of screening and vaccination programmes, play an important role in overall inequalities in health (Marmot et al, 1997), but there remains little understanding of why socioeconomic patterning of these behaviours persists and what can be done about it.

In 1995, Charlton and White proposed that the key links between socioeconomic position (SEP) and health-related behaviours are 'choice, autonomy and long termism' (Charlton and White, 1995, p 235). The concept they referred to as 'long termism' is more commonly termed 'time preference' or 'time perspective' and describes how individuals value and orientate themselves towards the future and how this influences their behaviour. The hypothesis that time preference and perspective may play a role in the link between socioeconomic factors and health-related behaviours is potentially important in terms of both understanding and developing interventions to reduce socioeconomic inequalities in health-related behaviours but remains under-researched.

Here I discuss how time preference and time perspective have been understood by both economists and psychologists, describe the theoretical reasons why time preference and perspective may be related to both SEP and health-related behaviours and briefly review the evidence relating to these relationships. I present a new conceptual model of the possible relationship between SEP, time preference and perspective, and health-related behaviours. I conclude that public health may have much to gain from integrating these economic and psychological concepts in its understanding of inequalities and that this is an area ripe for public health interventional development. Although previous reviews have collated evidence on the economic concept of time preference and health-related behaviours (Chapman, 2005), and the psychological concept of time perspective and alcoholism (Hulbert, 1988), no previous work has provided a comprehensive overview of both economic and psychological concepts and proposed that both may play a role in socioeconomic inequalities in health-related behaviours.

What are time preference and time perspective?

In general, it has been found that individuals would prefer to receive a gain today rather than in the future, and suffer a loss sometime in the future rather than today. Furthermore, the value of a future gain or loss, when looked at from the perspective of the present day, is somewhat less than that which will be realised once the future date is reached. Thus, for example, if individuals are asked to state what value of prize today would be equally attractive as a prize of £1,000 a year from today, the answer is, generally, somewhat less than £1,000. As the delay to the attainment of the prize increases, the current value of the delayed prize decreases, generally in a hyperbolic fashion (Mazur, 1987). This variation in preference for events according to time delay is referred to by economists as time preference and the rate at which the value of future prizes decreases over time the discount rate. The higher the discount rate, the more rapidly the value of delayed events decreases over time. Thus, increased time preference and discount rates indicate less preference for future events and more preference for present events (see Figure 2.1).

Figure 2.1: Current value of a £1,000 prize received after delays of up to 15 years according to four different discount rates (k=discount rate)

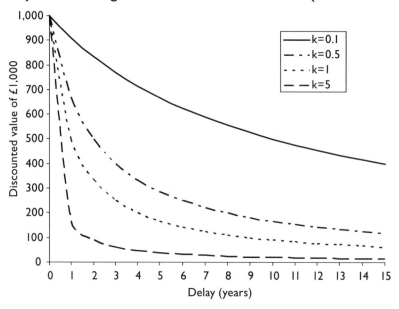

Although the phenomenon of time preference appears to be pervasive, discount rates vary between and within individuals according to the value of loss or gain considered (lower values are generally discounted more), the nature of that loss or gain (health is generally discounted less than money) and whether a loss or gain is considered (gains are generally discounted more than losses) (Baker et al, 2003). Given the known variability in time preference among individuals according to a number of factors, it is also possible that time preference varies according to both SEP and health-related behaviours.

In contrast to the economic focus on value over time, psychologists have focused on how often, and in what way, individuals consider past, present and future events when making behavioural decisions. A number of different concepts with a temporal dimension have been proposed (see Box 2.1). While all related in terms of their inclusion of a temporal perspective, these concepts are not all necessarily direct proxies of the time preference and perspective concept. While acknowledging the differences between the various terms listed in Box 2.1, I seek here to highlight the similarities, rather than the differences, and refer to the common time dimension of these psychological concepts using the general term 'time perspective'.

Time preference, time perspective and socioeconomic position

A number of studies have reported a relationship between SEP and both time preference and time perspective, finding that more affluent individuals tend to be more future orientated than more deprived individuals (Freire et al, 1980; Fuchs, 1980; Leigh, 1986; Nurmi, 1987; Lawrence, 1991; Green et al, 1996; Bosma et al, 1999; Peetsma, 2000; Wardle and Steptoe, 2003; Guiso and Paiella, 2004; Jaroni et al, 2004; Dom et al, 2006; Gurmankin-Levy et al, 2006). Instances where this relationship has not been found are predominantly case-control studies comparing current and never drug users (Kirby et al, 1999; Chesson and Viscusi, 2000; Petry, 2003; Reynolds et al, 2003; Kirby and Petry, 2004; Ohmura et al, 2005). As case-control studies are designed to identify differences and similarities between cases and controls, rather than associations between two continuous variables (Rothman, 1986), these findings are unlikely to be robust.

The main proposed explanation of time preference centres around uncertainty. The future is inherently uncertain and no future loss or gain can be absolutely guaranteed. As such, a future, and therefore uncertain, gain has less value than a current, and therefore almost certain, one (Freire et al, 1980). This explanation immediately raises the potential that time preference may be socioeconomically patterned. High-income occupations with permanent contracts and pension provision are frequently described as 'secure' in contrast to the relative insecurity and uncertainty of low incomes, temporary employment and reliance on state benefits. With money in the bank it begins to be possible to plan for the future. Without such savings and guaranteed income streams the future is uncertain

Box 2.1: Concepts from the psychological literature that propose a temporal dimension in behavioural decision making

Consideration of future consequences

> 'the extent to which people consider the potential distant outcomes of their current behaviours and the extent to which they are influenced by these potential outcomes' (Strathman et al, 1994)

Future orientation

> 'a positive belief in one's future' (Piko et al., 2005)

Time perspective

> 'the manner in which individuals and culture partition the flow of human experience into the distinct temporal categories of past, present and future' (Zimbardo et al, 1997)

> 'the often non-conscious process whereby the continual flow of personal and social experiences are decomposed or allocated into selected temporal categories or frames that help give order, coherence and meaning to those events' (Keough et al, 1999)

> 'provides the structure from which people select and pursue short-term or long-term goals' (Hamilton et al, 2003)

> 'a personality variable that refers to persons' time horizons. How far ahead in time do persons think about and plan their futures? To what degree do they use information about future outcomes in making decisions about current behaviour?' (Hodgins and Engel, 2002)

Delay of gratification

> 'an individual's ability to forfeit an immediate goal in order to obtain a preferred goal which is more distant in time' (Cuskelly et al, 2001)

Impulsivity

> 'acting without thinking' (Allen et al, 1998)

> 'quick decision making' (Allen et al, 1998)

> 'thinking about the present rather than the future' (Allen et al, 1998)

> 'it has been argued that most definitions of impulsivity can be related to a choice for a smaller more immediate reinforcer over a larger but more delayed reinforcer' (Allen et al, 1998)

Anticipatory regret

> 'the main psychological effects of the various worries that beset a decision maker before any losses actually materialize' (Richard et al, 1996)

and making firm plans becomes harder (Freire et al, 1980; Lawrence, 1991). The influence of income on security and ability to plan for the future strongly suggests that time preference and perspective should be socioeconomically patterned.

Educational attainment has also been used as a marker of time preference (Chaloupka, 1991; Huston and Finke, 2003). It is suggested that delaying entry to the workforce in order to take part in further education is an investment-like behaviour with low income in the short term being traded for higher income prospects in the longer term (Munasinghe and Sicherman, 2005). As educational attainment is also a key marker of SEP (Krieger et al, 1997; Galobardes et al, 2006), this provides a further theoretical link between SEP and time preference and perspective.

A number of authors have suggested that time preference and perspective are learned traits with children growing up in less structured environments and experiencing less predictability being more likely to develop high discount rates and less orientation towards the future (Frank, 1939; Zimbardo and Boyd, 1999; Petry, 2002). The preceding discussion suggests a number of reasons why less affluent families may provide less certain environments. Given that SEP tracks through the lifecourse, with children tending to maintain the relative social position of the families they were born into throughout adulthood (Graham, 2002), this provides further reason to believe that there may be a persistent relationship between SEP and time preference and perspective.

Lastly, children from more affluent families may gain a more developed sense of the future because their futures are, to some degree, more planned than children from less affluent families. Affluent children may be more likely than deprived children to be expected to finish school and attend university – providing a clear plan for their future into their early twenties. In contrast, children from more deprived families may face expectations to leave school in their mid-teens and find a job – providing a clear plan only into the mid- or late teens (Nurmi, 1991).

Time preference, time perspective and health-related behaviours

Many health-promoting messages appeal to a desire to make the future better – or at least more healthy – encouraging us to adopt healthy behaviours now in order to safeguard our health in the future (Rakowski, 1986; Orbell and Hagger, 2006). Similarly, many health-related behaviours involve a trade-off between immediate pleasure and potential future health benefits (Fuchs, 1980; Finke, 2000; Piko et al, 2005). For example, eating a healthy diet involves avoiding pleasurable, but unhealthy foods in the short term and taking part in a regular exercise programme involves devoting time, energy and, in some cases, money in the short term – both in order to reduce the risk of a number of chronic diseases in the long term. Despite some current attempts to make healthy behaviours 'fashionable' and therefore attractive in the short term, the reality is that many behaviours have to be pursued for prolonged periods of time in order to bring health benefits and those benefits are not certain. Thus, a rational decision to take part in healthy behaviours – for the purpose of health benefit – requires that value is placed on potential health benefit at some point in the future. Hence, it is highly plausible that time preference and perspective play a role in the decision to take part in healthy behaviours.

Although there is strong theoretical reason why time preference and perspective may be important in determining many different health behaviours, the majority of the empirical evidence on the ability of time preference and perspective to predict health behaviours has focused on addictive behaviours. Many studies have now reported that people who use substances such as heroin, cocaine, alcohol and tobacco in an addictive manner have higher discount rates than individuals who do not (Hornik, 1990; Madden et al, 1997; Vuchinich and Simpson, 1998; Bickel et al, 1999; Bretteville-Jensen, 1999; Kirby et al, 1999; Mitchell, 1999; Petry and Casarella, 1999; Chen, 2001; Petry, 2001, 2002, 2003; Odum et al, 2002; Baker et al, 2003; Coffey et al, 2003; Sato and Ohkusa, 2003; Kirby and Petry, 2004; Reynolds et al, 2004; Ohmura et al, 2005; Dom et al, 2006). In addition, there is consistent evidence of a cross-sectional relationship between psychological measures of time perspective and use of addictive substances (Sattler and Pflugrath, 1970; Alvos et al, 1993; Businelle, 1996; Allen et al, 1998; Petry et al, 1998; Vuchinich and Simpson, 1998; Keough et al, 1999; Chen, 2001; Klingemann, 2001; Wills et al, 2001; Levy and Earleywine, 2004; Robbins and Bryan, 2004; Peters et al, 2005; Piko et al, 2005), with only two known studies failing to report the predicted relationship (Murphy and DeWolfe, 1985-86; Chesson and Viscusi, 2000).

Much less work has explored the relationship between measures of time preference and perspective and non-addictive health-related behaviours. While condom use and other safer sexual practices appear to be associated with more orientation towards the future (Rothspan and Read, 1996; Agnew and Loving, 1998; Dorr et al, 1999; Aronowitz and Morrison-Beedy, 2004; Bryan et al, 2004; Appleby et al, 2005), time preference was not strongly associated with acceptance of an influenza vaccine or adherence with hypertension or cholesterol medication prescriptions (Chapman and Coups, 1999; Chapman et al, 2001). Other behaviours such as fruit and vegetable intake and regular physical activity are inconsistently related to measures of time preference and perspective (Mahon and Yarcheski, 1994; Mahon et al, 1997, 2000; Finke, 2000; Hamilton et al, 2003; Huston and Finke, 2003; Wardle and Steptoe, 2003; Nagin and Pogarsky, 2004) but few of these studies used well-established, or validated, measures of time preference or perspective and behavioural measures were frequently crude and sample sizes small.

Gaps in the literature, methodological problems and next steps

The evidence reviewed thus far, along with the well-established relationships between SEP and both addictive and non-addictive health-related behaviours, is summarised in a new conceptual model shown in Figure 2.2. In this figure, solid arrows represent established relationships and the dotted arrow represents a hypothesised relationship that may be an area of fruitful future investigation.

Figure 2.2: Hypothesised pathways linking SEP, time preference and perspective, and health-related behaviours

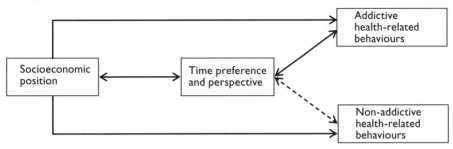

There is substantial evidence that time preference and perspective are socioeconomically patterned and that addictive behaviours are associated with increased time preference and less orientation towards the future. Given the strength of the evidence, these relationships are represented with solid arrows in Figure 2.2. While there is good theoretical reason to believe that other, non-addictive, health-related behaviours are associated with time preference and perspective, this relationship has received little attention in the literature. Due to the current absence of evidence on this relationship (rather than evidence of absence of a relationship), it is represented by a dotted arrow in Figure 2.2. As there is good evidence (not reviewed here) that SEP is a causal determinant of health-related behaviours, these relationships are shown with unidirectional arrows in Figure 2.2. However, the direction of causation, if any, between SEP and time preference and perspective, and between time preference and perspective and health-related behaviours is not known and these relationships are, therefore, shown with bidirectional arrows in Figure 2.2.

The current gaps in the literature highlighted by Figure 2.2, along with a number of others, are now discussed in turn.

Time preference, time perspective and socioeconomic inequalities in health-related behaviours

Although all of the individual relationships shown in Figure 2.2 have been subject to at least some empirical testing, few attempts have been made to study the whole pathway. In the cases where time preference and perspective have been investigated as potential mediators of the relationship between SEP and health-related behaviours, it has been found that time preference or time perspective statistically accounts for some, but not all, of the relationship between SEP and health-related behaviours (Fuchs, 1980; Hornik, 1990; Keough et al, 1999; Picone et al, 2004; Appleby et al, 2005). Further work using well-established measures of time preference and perspective, SEP and health-related behaviours is, therefore, required to determine if a causal pathway exists linking SEP and health-related behaviours through time preference and perspective.

Lack of longitudinal data

To date, a substantial proportion of published research on time preference and perspective in relation to health behaviours has relied on case-control studies of substance users versus non-users where time preference or perspective is measured after behavioural patterns are well established. Although these studies provide useful preliminary evidence, they cannot provide any evidence on causality. Furthermore, even if a causal association is assumed, case-control studies provide no information of the direction of causality – is time preference a constant factor within individuals that determines their behaviours, or do individuals alter their time preference in order to be consistent with the behaviours they currently perform? The existing, scant, longitudinal data provide evidence for both possibilities (Henik and Domino, 1975; Reynolds et al, 2003, 2004).

Further, rigorous longitudinal work that explores the effect of behaviour change on time preference and perspective, and the effect of time preference and perspective on behaviour change, will be necessary to help establish a causal relationship and the direction of causality between time preference and perspective and health-related behaviours.

Problems with definition and measurement

Along with the wide variety of concepts that have some relation to the time preference and perspective concept (Box 2.1) there has been wide variation in methods of measurement. A number of different choice tasks (Green et al, 1994; Chesson and Viscusi, 2000; Chapman et al, 2001), personality inventories (Strathman et al, 1994; Zimbardo and Boyd, 1999) and other tasks (Freire et al, 1980; Leigh, 1986) have been developed that purport to measure time preference, time perspective and related concepts. While some of the personality inventories have been subject to ample psychometric testing (Strathman et al, 1994; Zimbardo et al, 1997; Zimbardo and Boyd, 1999; D'Alessio et al, 2003), and money choice tasks appear to produce results in line with a variety of theoretical predictions (Mazur, 1987), without a clear conceptualisation of the phenomenon under study it is almost impossible to confirm construct validity.

Other proxies that have been proposed and used as measures of time preference or time perspective include smoking (Chaloupka, 1991; Munasinghe and Sicherman, 2000; Fersterer and Winter-Ebmer, 2003; Huston and Finke, 2003; Munasinghe and Sicherman, 2005), educational attainment (Chaloupka, 1991; Huston and Finke, 2003), spending patterns (Barsky et al, 1997; Komlos et al, 2004; Picone et al, 2004) and predicted longevity (Wardle and Steptoe, 2003; Nagin and Pogarsky, 2004; Picone et al, 2004). However, these all have limitations in the context of socioeconomic inequalities in health-related behaviours – educational attainment is a common marker of SEP (Krieger et al, 1997; Galobardes et al, 2006), spending patterns and longevity are strongly associated with SEP (Drever and Whitehead, 1997) and smoking is a key health-related behaviour. The development of both an integrated definition of the concept of time preference and time perspective, and a measurement instrument that incorporates both economic and psychological perspectives, is therefore required to enable good-quality and policy-relevant, multidisciplinary work to be performed in this area.

Developing health-promotion interventions

From a public health perspective, the finding that time preference and perspective play a role in mediating the relationship between SEP and health-related behaviours is only of interest if it can be used to help promote wider uptake of healthy behaviours – particularly among individuals from the most deprived groups. Two approaches have been taken to making use of time preference and perspective in the area of health-promotion interventions.

On the basis that there is some evidence of a cross-sectional relationship between health behaviours and time preference and perspective, a few researchers have attempted to promote healthy behaviours by manipulating time perspective. These manipulations generally take the form of asking participants to focus on the future benefits of healthy behaviour, or the negative thoughts they may experience after engaging in unhealthy behaviours, and have led to some short-term success in behavioural change (Richard et al, 1996; Murgraff et al, 1999; Hall and Fong, 2003). Longer-term studies are required to determine if such interventions lead to sustained alteration in both time preference and perspective and behaviour.

A second body of work has proposed that the effectiveness of health-promoting messages may vary with an individual's time preference or perspective. There is some evidence that those with more future-orientated time perspectives respond better to traditional health-promoting interventions that focus on future benefits of behaviour while those with more present-orientated time perspectives respond better to messages that stress the short-term benefits of behaviour (Orbell et al, 2004; Ouellette et al, 2005; Orbell and Hagger, 2006). The obvious conclusion is that tailoring health-promotion messages to the time perspective of the subject may be more effective than a 'one-size-fits-all' approach – similar to the tailoring of health-promotion messages to individuals' stage of change proposed by the transtheoretical model (Prochaska and DiClemente, 1982).

Conclusions

In this chapter I have proposed that attitudes towards the future, encapsulated in the concepts of time preference and perspective, may play a role in mediating the pervasive link between SEP and health-related behaviours. Strong theoretical reasons why time preference and perspective should be both associated with SEP and predictive of health-related behaviours have been presented. The evidence reviewed here confirms a link between SEP and time preference and perspective and between addictive behaviours and time preference and perspective. Further work is required to confirm that time preference and perspective are associated with non-addictive health-related behaviours and that time preference and perspective are on the causal pathway between SEP and health-related behaviours. Some preliminary work suggests that interventions to alter time perspective or tailor health-promotion interventions according to recipients' time preference may be effective in achieving behaviour change. Public health specialists may have much to gain by integrating these psychological and economic concepts into their understanding of socioeconomic inequalities in health and health-related behaviours.

Acknowledgements

Many thanks to Professors Cam Donaldson, Martin White and Andrew Steptoe for providing critical comments on previous drafts of this chapter. The author is supported by a UK MRC Special Training Fellowship in Health Services and Health of the Public Research.

References

Acheson, D. (1998) *Report of the independent inquiry into inequalities in health*, London: The Stationery Office.

Agnew, C.R. and Loving, T.J. (1998) 'Future time orientation and condom use: attitudes, intentions, and behavior', *Journal of Social Behavior and Personality* 13: 755-64.

Allen, T.J., Moeller, G., Rhoades, H.M. and Cherek, D.R. (1998) 'Impulsivity and history of drug dependence' *Drug and Alcohol Dependence* 50: 137-45.

Alvarez-Dardet, C. and Ashton, J. (2005) 'News scoop–hold the front page: "poverty damages health"', *Journal of Epidemiology and Community Health* 59: 89.

Alvos, L., Gregson, R. and Ross, M. (1993) 'Future time perspective in current and previous injecting drug users', *Drug and Alcohol Dependence* 31: 193-7.

Appleby, P., Marks, G., Ayala, A., Miller, L., Murphy, S. and Mansergh, G. (2005) 'Consideration of future consequences and unprotected anal intercourse among men who have sex with men', *Journal of Homosexuality* 50: 119-33.

Arblaster, L., Lambert, M., Entwistle, V., Forster, M., Fullerton, D., Sheldon, T. and Watt, I. (1996) 'A systematic review of the effectiveness of health service interventions aimed at reducing inequalities in health', *Journal of Health Service Research Policy* 1: 93-103.

Aronowitz, T. and Morrison-Beedy, D. (2004) 'Resilience to risk-taking behaviours in impoverished African American girls: the role of mother-daughter connections', *Research in Nursing and Health* 27: 29-39.

Baker, F., Johnson, M. and Bickel, W. (2003) 'Delay discounting in current and never-before cigarette smokers: similarities and differences across commodity, sign, and magnitude', *Journal of Abnormal Psychology* 112: 382-92.

Barsky, R., Juster, F., Kimball, M. and Shapiro, M. (1997) 'Preference parameters and behavioural heterogeneity: an experimental approach in the Health and Retirement Study', *The Quarterly Journal of Economics* 112: 538-78.

Bickel, W.K., Odum, A.L. and Madden, G.J. (1999) 'Impulsivity and cigarette smoking: delay discounting in current, never, and ex-smokers', *Psychopharmacology* 146: 447-54.

Bosma, H., Van De Mheen, H. and Mackenbach, J. (1999) 'Social class in childhood and general health in adulthood: questionnaire study of contribution of psychological attributes', *British Medical Journal* 318: 18-22.

Bretteville-Jensen, A. (1999) 'Addiction and discounting', *Journal of Health Economics*, 18: 393-407.

Bryan, A., Aiken, L. and West, S. (2004) 'HIV/STD risk among incarcerated adolescents: optimism about the future and self-esteem as predictors of condom use self-efficacy', *Journal of Applied Social Psychology* 34: 912-36.

Businelle, M. (1996) 'Heavy smokers choose large, immediate rewards with large penalties on a simulated task of gambling', Thesis, Department of Psychology, University of Southwestern Louisiana, Louisiana, LA.

Chaloupka, F. (1991) 'Rational addictive behaviour and cigarette smoking', *Journal of Political Economy* 99: 723-42.

Chapman, G. (2005) 'Short-term cost for long-term benefit: time preference and cancer control', *Health Psychology* 24: 541-8.

Chapman, G. and Coups, E. (1999) 'Time preferences and preventive health behaviour', *Medical Decision Making* 19: 307-14.

Chapman, G., Brewer, N., Coups, E., Brownlee, S. and Leventhal, H. (2001) 'Value for the future and preventive health behaviour', *Journal of Experimental Psychology: Applied* 7: 235-50.

Charlton, B. and White, M. (1995) 'Living on the margin: a salutogenic model for socioeconomic differentials in health', *Public Health* 109: 235-43.

Chen, K. (2001) 'Time preference and cigarette smoking in adolescents', *Journal of Addictive Diseases* 20: 134.

Chesson, H. and Viscusi, W. (2000) 'The heterogeneity of time-risk tradeoffs', *Journal of Behavioural Decision Making* 13: 251-8.

Coffey, S., Gudleski, G., Saladin, M. and Brady, K. (2003) 'Impulsivity and rapid discounting of delayed hypothetical rewards in cocaine-dependent individuals', *Experimental and Clinical Psychopharmacology* 11: 18-25.

Cuskelly, M., Einam, M. and Jobling, A. (2001) 'Delay of gratification in young adults with Down syndrome', *Down Syndrome Research and Practice* 7: 60-7.

D'Alessio, M., Guarino, A., Pascalis, V. and Zimbardo, P.G. (2003) 'Testing Zimbardo's Stanford Time Perspective Inventory (STPI) short form: an Italian study', *Time and Society* 12: 333-47.

Dom, G., D'haene, P., Hulstijn, W. and Sabbe, B. (2006) 'Impulsivity in abstinent early- and late-onset alcoholics: difference in self-report measure and a discounting task', *Addiction* 101: 50-9.

Dorr, N., Krueckeberg, S., Strathman, A. and Wood, M. (1999) 'Psychosocial correlates of voluntary HIV antibody testing in college students', *AIDS Education and Prevention* 11: 14-27.

Drever, F. and Whitehead, M. (eds) (1997) *Health inequalities decennial supplement* London: The Stationery Office.

Fersterer, J. and Winter-Ebmer, R. (2003) 'Smoking, discount rates, and returns to education', *Economics of Education Review* 22(6): 561-6.

Finke, M. (2000) 'Did the Nutrition Labelling and Education Act affect food choice in the United States? American Consumer and the Changing Structure of the Food System conference', Economic Research Service, USDA, Arlington, VA, 3-5 May.

Frank, L. (1939)'Time perspectives', *Journal of Social Philosophy* 4: 293-312.

Freire, E., Gorman, B. and Wessman, E. (1980)'Temporal span, delay of gratification, and children's socioeconomic status', *Journal of Genetic Psychology* 137: 247-55.

Fuchs, V. (1980) *Time preference and health: an exploratory study*, Cambridge, MA, National Bureau of Economic Research.

Galobardes, B., Shaw, M., Lawlor, D.A., Lynch, J.W. and Davey Smith, G. (2006) 'Indicators of socioeconomic position (part 1)', *Journal of Epidemiology and Community Health* 60: 7-12.

Graham, H. (2002) 'Building an inter-disciplinary science of health inequalities: the example of lifecourse research', *Social Science and Medicine* 55: 2005-16.

Green, L., Fry, A. and Myerson, J. (1994) 'Discounting of delayed rewards: a life-span comparison', *Psychological Science* 5: 33-6.

Green, L., Myerson, J., Lichtman, D., Rosen, S. and Fry, A. (1996) 'Temporal discounting in choice between delayed rewards: the role of age and income', *Psychology and Aging* 11: 79-84.

Guiso, L. and Paiella, M. (2004) 'The role of risk aversion in predicting individual behaviour', Latin American Meeting of the Econometrics Society, Santiago, Chile, 28–30 July.

Gunning-Schepers, L. and Gepkens, A. (1996) 'Reviews of interventions to reduce social inequalities in health: research and policy implications', *Health Education Research* 55: 226-38.

Gurmankin-Levy, A., Micco, E., Putt, M. and Armstrong, K. (2006) 'Value for the future and breast cancer preventive health behavior', *Cancer Epidemiology Biomarkers & Prevention* 15: 955-60.

Hall, P. and Fong, G. (2003) 'The effects of a brief time perspective intervention for increasing physical activity among young adults', *Psychology and Health* 18: 685-706.

Hamilton, J., Kives, K., Micevski, V. and Grace, S. (2003) 'Time perspective and health-promoting behavior in a cardiac rehabilitation population', *Behavioral Medicine* 28: 132-9.

Henik, W. and Domino, G. (1975) 'Alterations in future time perspective in heroin addicts', *Journal of Clinical Psychology* 31: 557-64.

Hodgins, D. and Engel, A. (2002) 'Future time perspective in pathological gamblers', *Journal of Nervous and Mental Disease* 190: 775-9.

Hornik, J. (1990) 'Time preference, psychographics, and smoking behaviour', *Journal of Health Care Marketing* 10: 36-46.

Hulbert, R. (1988) 'Time perspective, time attitude, and time orientation in alcoholism: a review', *The International Journal of Addiction* 23: 279-98.

Huston, S. and Finke, M. (2003) 'Diet choice and the role of time preference', *Journal of Consumer Affairs* 37: 143-60.

Jaroni, J., Wright, S., Lerman, C. and Epstein, L. (2004) 'Relationship between education and delay discounting in smokers', *Addictive Behaviours* 29: 1171-5.

Keough, K.A., Zimbardo, P.G. and Boyd, J.N. (1999) 'Who's smoking, drinking, and using drugs? Time perspective as a predictor of substance use', *Basic and Applied Social Psychology* 2: 149-64.

Kirby, K. and Petry, N. (2004) 'Heroin and cocaine abusers have higher discount rates for delayed rewards than alcoholics or non-drug-using controls', *Society for the Study of Addiction* 99: 461-71.

Kirby, K., Petry, N. and Bickel, W. (1999) 'Heroin addicts have higher discount rates for delayed rewards than non-drug-using controls', *Journal of Experimental Psychology: General* 128: 78-87.

Klingemann, H. (2001) 'The time game: temporal perspectives of patients and staff in alcohol and drug treatment', *Time and Society* 10: 303-28.

Komlos, J., Smith, P. and Bogin, B. (2004) 'Obesity and the rate of time preference: is there a connection?', *Journal of Biosocial Science* 36: 209-19.

Krieger, N., Williams, D. and Moss, N. (1997) 'Measuring social class in US public health research: concepts, methodologies and guidelines', *Annual Review of Public Health* 18: 341-78.

Lawrence, E. (1991) 'Poverty and the rate of time preference: evidence from panel data', *Journal of Political Economy'* 99: 54-77.

Leigh, J. (1986) Accounting for tastes: correlates of risk and time preferences', *Journal of Post Keynesian Economics* 9: 17-31.

Levy, B. and Earleywine, M. (2004) 'Discriminating reinforcement expectancies for studying from future time perspective in the prediction of drinking problems', *Addictive Behaviours* 29: 181-90.

Mackenbach, J., Kunst, A., Cavelaars, E., Groenhof, F. and Geurts, J. (1997) 'Socioeconomic inequalities in morbidity and mortality in Western Europe'. *The Lancet* 349: 1655-9.

Madden, G., Petry, N., Badger, G. and Bickel, W. (1997) 'Impulsive and self-control choices in opioid-dependent patients and non-drug-using control participants: drug and monetary rewards', *Experimental and Clinical Psychopharmachology* 5: 256-62.

Mahon, N. and Yarcheski, T. (1994) 'Future time perspective and positive health practices in adolescents', *Perceptual and Motor Skills* 79: 395-8.

Mahon, N., Yarcheski, T. and Yarcheski, A. (1997) 'Future time perspective and positive health practices in young adults: an extension', *Perceptual and Motor Skills* 84: 1299-304.

Mahon, N., Yarcheski, T. and Yarcheski, A. (2000) 'Future time perspective and positive health practices among young adolescents: a further extension', *Perceptual and Motor Skills* 90: 166-8.

Marmot, M., Bosma, H., Hemingway, H., Brunner, E. and Stansfeld, S. (1997) 'Contribution of job control and other risk factors to social variations in coronary heart disease incidence', *The Lancet* 350: 235-9.

Mazur, J.E. (1987) 'An adjusting procedure for studying delayed reinforcement', in M.L. Commons, J.E. Mazur, J.A. Nevin and H. Rachlin (eds) *Quantitative analysis of behaviour: The effect of delay and intervening events on reinforcement value.* Hillsdale, NJ, Erlbaum Associates: 55-73.

Mitchell, S.H. (1999) 'Measures of impulsivity in cigarette smokers and non-smokers', *Psychopharmacology* 146: 455-64.

Munasinghe, L. and Sicherman, N. (2000) *Why do dancers smoke? Time preference, occupational choice, and wage growth*, NBER Working Paper Series, Cambridge, MA: National Bureau of Economic Research, www.nber.org/papers/w7542.pdf

Munasinghe, L. and Sicherman, N. (2005) *Wage dynamics and unobserved heterogeneity: Time preference or learning ability?*, NBER Working Paper Series Cambridge, MA: National Bureau of Economic Research, www.nber.org/papers/w11031.pdf

Murgraff, V., McDermoot, M., White, D. and Phillips, K. (1999) 'Regret is what you get: the effects of manipulating anticipated affect and time perspective on risky single-occasion drinking', *Alcohol and Alcoholism* 34: 590-600.

Murphy, T. and DeWolfe, A. (1985-86) 'Future time perspective in alcoholics process and reactive schizophrenics, and normals', *International Journal of Addiction* 20: 1815-22.

Nagin, D. and Pogarsky, G. (2004) 'Time and punishment: delayed consequences and criminal behaviour', *Journal of Quantitative Criminology* 20: 295-317.

Nurmi, J. (1987) 'Age, sex, social class, and quality of family interaction as determinants of adolescents' future orientation: a developmental task interpretation', *Adolescence* 22: 978-91.

Nurmi, J. (1991) 'How do adolescents see their future? A review of the development of future orientation and planning', *Developmental Review* 11: 1-59.

Odum, A.L., Madden, G.J. and Bickel, W.K. (2002) 'Discounting of delayed health gains and losses by current, never- and ex-smokers of cigarettes', *Nicotine and Tobacco Research* 4: 295-303.

Ohmura, Y., Takahashi, T. and Kitamura, N. (2005) 'Discounting delayed and probabilistic monetary gains and losses by smokers of cigarettes', *Psychopharmacology* 182: 508-15.

Orbell, S. and Hagger, M. (2006) 'Temporal framing and the decision to take part in Type 2 diabetes screening: effects of individual differences in consideration of future consequences on persuasion', *Health Psychology* 25(4): 537-48.

Orbell, S., Perugini, M. and Rakow, T. (2004) 'Individual differences in sensitivity to health communications: consideration of future consequences', *Health Psychology* 23: 388-96.

Ouellette, J., Hessling, R., Gibbons, F., Reis-Bergan, M. and Gerrard, M. (2005) 'Using images to increase exercise behavior: prototypes versus possible selves', *Personality and Social Psychology Bulletin* 31: 610-20.

Peetsma, T. (2000) 'Future time perspective as a predictor of school investment', *Scandinavian Journal of Educational Research* 44: 178-92.

Peters, R., Tortolero, S., Johnson, R., Addy, R., Markham, C., Escobar-Chaves, L., Lewis, H. and Yacoubian, G. (2005) 'The relationship between future orientation and street substance use among Texas alternative school students', *American Journal of Addictions* 14: 478-85.

Petry, N. (2001) 'Delay discounting of money and alcohol in actively using alcoholics, currently abstinent alcoholics, and controls', *Psychopharmacology* 154: 243-50.

Petry, N. (2002) 'Discounting of delayed rewards in substance abusers: relationship to antisocial personality disorder', *Psychopharmacology* 162: 425-32.

Petry, N. (2003) 'Discounting of money, health, and freedom in substance abusers and controls', *Drug and Alcohol Dependence* 71: 133-41.

Petry, N. and Casarella, T. (1999) 'Excessive discounting of delayed rewards in substance abusers with gambling problems', *Drug and Alcohol Dependence* 56: 25-32.

Petry, N., Wk, B. and Arnett, M. (1998) 'Shortened time horizons and insensitivity to future consequences in heroin addicts', *Addiction* 93: 729-38.

Picone, G., Sloan, F. and Taylor, D. (2004) 'Effects of risk and time preference and expected longevity on demand for medical tests', *Journal of Risk & Uncertainty* 28(1): 39-53.

Piko, B. F., Luszczynska, A., Gibbons, F. X. and Tekozel, M. (2005) 'A culture-based study of personal and social influences of adolescent smoking', *European Journal of Public Health* 15: 393-8.

Prochaska, J. and Diclemente, C. (1982) 'Transtheoretical therapy: toward a more integrative model of change', *Psychotherapy: Theory, Research and Practice* 19: 276-88.

Rakowski, W. (1986) 'Future time perspective: applications to the health context of later adulthood', *American Behavioural Scientist* 29: 730-45.

Reynolds, B., Karraker, K., Horn, K. and Richards, J. (2003) 'Delay and probability discounting as related to different stages of adolescent smoking and non-smoking', *Science Direct* 64: 333-44.

Reynolds, B., Richards, J.B., Horn, K. and Karraker, K. (2004) 'Delay discounting and probability discounting as related to cigarette smoking status in adults', *Behavioural Processes* 65: 35-42.

Richard, R., De Vries, N. and Van Der Pligt, J. (1996) 'Anticipated affect and behavioral choice', *Basic and Applied Social Psychology* 18: 111-29.

Robbins, R. and Bryan, A. (2004) 'Relationships between future orientation, impulsive sensation seeking, and risk behavior among adjudicated adolescents', *Journal of Adolescent Research* 19: 428-45.

Rothman, K. (1986) *Modern epidemiology*, Boston, MA: Little, Brown.

Rothspan, S. and Read, S. (1996) 'Present versus future time perspective and HIV risk among heterosexual college students', *Health Psychology* 15: 131-4.

Sato, M. and Ohkusa, Y. (2003) 'The relationship between smoking initiation and time discount factor, risk aversion and information', *Applied Economics Letters* 10: 287-9.

Sattler, J. and Pflugrath, J. (1970) 'Future-time perspective in alcoholics and normals', *Quarterly Journal of Studies in Alcohol* 31: 839-50.

Strathman, A., Gleicher, F., Boninger, D.S. and Edwards, C.S. (1994) 'The consideration of future consequences: weighing immediate and distant outcomes of behavior', *Journal of Personality and Social Psychology* 66: 742-52.

Vuchinich, R. and Simpson, C. (1998) 'Hyperbolic temporal discounting in social drinkers and problem drinkers', *Experimental and Clinical Psychopharmachology* 6: 292-305.

Wardle, J. and Steptoe, A. (2003) 'Socioeconomic differences in attitudes and beliefs about healthy lifestyles', *Journal of Epidemiology and Community Health* 57: 440-3.

Wills, T., Sandy, J. and Yaeger, A. (2001) 'Time perspective and early-onset substance use: a model based on stress-coping theory', *Psychology of Addictive Behaviour* 15: 118-25.

Zimbardo, P. G. and Boyd, J. N. (1999) 'Putting time in perspective: a valid, reliable individual-differences metric', *Journal of Personality and Social Psychology* 77: 1271-88.

Zimbardo, P., Keough, K. and Boyd, J. (1997) 'Present time perspective as a predictor of risky driving', *Experimental and Clinical Psychopharmacology* 23: 1007-23.

THREE

Examination of the built environment and prevalence of obesity: neighbourhood characteristics, food purchasing venues, green space and distribution of Body Mass Index

Tamara Dubowitz, Theresa L. Osypuk and Kristen Kurland

Introduction and background

Obesity has become an epidemic in the US and it is poised to become the nation's leading health problem. Sixty-five per cent of the US population is either overweight or obese. However, the condition is not evenly distributed along racial, socioeconomic or gender lines. The prevalence of adult overweight and obesity is higher among Hispanics and African Americans than among non-Hispanic white people (Flegal et al, 2002). African Americans have the highest obesity rates and have also experienced the steepest increases in Body Mass Index (BMI) over time (McTigue et al, 2002; Schoenborn et al, 2002; Denney, et al, 2004). Among Hispanics, African Americans and white people, women are more likely to be overweight and obese than men (Flegal et al, 2002; Hedley et al, 2004). Rates of overweight are higher for adults of low socioeconomic status (SES) (Drewnowski and Specter, 2004). There is strong evidence that women living below the poverty level are much more likely to be overweight or obese than women with higher incomes (Sobal and Stunkard, 1989; Stunkard, 1996; Chang and Lauderdale, 2005). Although the evidence for men is not so clear cut, there is evidence of a weak inverse relationship between income and obesity for white non-Hispanic men (Chang and Lauderdale, 2005).

Rapidly changing diets and reduced physical activity levels have led to a marked increase in the prevalence of diet-related chronic diseases in both developed and developing countries (Popkin, 1998, 2003). What circumstances have led to this trend? And why and how have disparities in obesity prevalence become so profound? This chapter seeks to address these questions by focusing on the relationship between obesity and its social context. We focus on the built and social residential environment of individuals, with the implicit understanding that there are myriad factors on biological and social levels that contribute towards obesity and its related consequences (for example, diabetes and cardiovascular disease). However, this chapter highlights how the residential environment of individuals can frame their health-related behaviours related to obesity, specifically diet and physical activity. We use the example of Pittsburgh, Pennsylvania, to examine the distribution of obesity within the city in relation to (1) the green space environment, (2) the distribution of food purchasing venues and (3) the sociodemographic characteristics of neighbourhoods within the city.

There is growing evidence that demonstrates that the 'physical' or 'built environment' plays an important role in health, especially with respect to obesity (Booth et al, 2005). The built environment may promote individual energy balance through fostering or discouraging certain health behaviours, including (but not limited to) diet and physical activity. Broadly, research has focused on:

- access to amenities;
- physical features of the environment and the degree of urbanisation;
- the reputation of the neighbourhood and resulting feelings of safety and crime;
- neighbourhood aesthetics; and
- the social organisation of the local community (Poortinga, 2006).

This chapter presents an overview of how socioeconomic and racial residential segregation foster neighbourhood inequality, particularly with respect to obesity. We also present evidence linking neighbourhoods to diet, exercise and obesity and follow this with our conceptual model guiding our interest in looking at characteristics of the social and built environment and prevalence of overweight and obesity using data from Pittsburgh as a case study.

Residential segregation and obesity

Although there are multiple mechanisms that operate at the level of individual lifestyle choices, there is increasing evidence that neighbourhood resources condition and restrict those choices (Berkman and Kawachi, 2000). Racial minority groups, especially black people, experience high levels of residential segregation across metropolitan areas in the US. Segregation by SES, although also present, is lower than segregation by race (Iceland et al, 2005). Residential segregation has been deemed a fundamental cause of racial health disparities, because of the effect of living in impoverished neighbourhoods, and the powerful effect of segregation influencing later life socioeconomic position (SEP) advancement – for example through lower-quality schools and constraints on access to other services. Residential segregation may influence health and obesity disparities through neighbourhood quality pathways, lifecourse SEP advancement or blocked advancement, as well as health behaviour pathways that might relate to coping (Collins and Williams, 2001; Acevedo-Garcia et al, 2003). For instance, one recent study has found that black people living in more segregated metropolitan areas exhibit higher rates of obesity (Chang, 2006).

As articulated by Schulz and colleagues (2002), segregation influences access to social and material resources that are directly associated with health at both individual and neighbourhood levels. Racially and socioeconomically segregated neighbourhoods are also more likely to be impoverished, and more likely to be high in violent crime (Massey, 1995; Sampson et al, 1997). Dangerous neighbourhood environments, or the perception of unsafe environments, may be linked to lower rates of exercise (Molnar et al, 2004). Fear of crime or difficulty monitoring children's behaviour might lead to parents' keeping children inside instead of them participating in outdoor physical activity. Thus, neighbourhood poverty – within the context of segregation – may influence health through a number of mechanisms, including access to services and amenities, feelings of safety, social cohesion and neighbourhood aesthetics, as well as the food and green space environment.

Neighbourhoods and diet

Better diet may result either from improved access to healthy foods or from reduced exposure to unhealthy food outlets, that is, fast foods, which are systematically patterned across different types of neighbourhoods. For instance, low-income and minority ethnic neighbourhoods have higher concentrations of fast-food establishments (Morland et al, 2002; Block et al, 2004; Moore and Diez Roux, 2006). Brownell has researched the 'toxic food environment' in the US, demonstrating that availability of foods high in fat and sugar, vending machines that often store less nutritious foods, fast-food outlets, large serving sizes and heavy marketing by the food industry all contribute to less healthy food choice (Brownell, 2005).

The neighbourhoods and diet literature has primarily examined dietary patterns by neighbourhood SES. Morland and colleagues (2002) found disparities in food availability by both income and racial characteristics of neighbourhoods; their findings demonstrated more supermarkets in wealthier neighbourhoods compared to poorer neighbourhoods, and four times more supermarkets located in white neighbourhoods compared to black neighbourhoods. Residence in more affluent neighbourhoods is associated with increased intake of fruit and vegetables (Morland et al, 2002; Shohaimi et al, 2004), whereas residence in lower SES areas (as measured by education level and poverty) is associated with lower fruit and vegetable consumption (Diez Roux et al, 1999; Morland et al, 2002).

Research has also demonstrated that unequal distribution of the quality and number of food purchasing venues within neighbourhoods is associated with diet. In a study of low-income African American women, Zenk and colleagues (2005) found that those women who purchased food at supermarkets and specialty stores consumed fruit and vegetables more often, on average, than those shopping at independent grocers. Perceived selection and quality of produce was also associated with fruit and vegetable intake, after adjusting for the type and location of the store in addition to age, per capita income and educational status. These results demonstrated that women with higher per capita incomes were more likely to shop at supermarkets than at other grocers, which in turn was associated with intake (Zenk et al, 2005).

However, understanding how residential neighbourhoods might impact diet involves recognition that individuals, within the context of their neighbourhoods, have multiple influences such as, for example, work schedule, childcare responsibilities and family structure (that is, whether a single-parent or a couple household) (Dubowitz et al, 2005). Any and/or all of these factors could moderate (or interact with) the effect of neighbourhood factors. One challenge is to disentangle the links between neighbourhoods and the individuals who inhabit them. For example, poorer neighbourhoods with fewer resources are also (by definition) populated by individuals with fewer resources, in comparison to richer neighbourhoods. Thus, individuals, or households, with fewer resources might have less time and flexibility than those individuals or households with greater resources. And therefore, neighbourhood factors, such as location and type of grocery stores and/or location and types of food-serving places, might have differing influences on different groups of people in terms of food purchasing, preparation and diet (Dubowitz et al, 2005).

Neighbourhoods and physical activity

Several disciplines, for instance transportation, urban design and planning disciplines, have developed conceptual and empirical work on how neighbourhoods influence physical activity, especially with regard to walking and cycling (Saelens et al, 2003). Factors that contribute towards physical activity within the built environment include, but are not limited to, the availability of facilities for physical activity, the distance between place of residence and exercise facilities and the perceived quality and safety of the environment in which physical activity might occur (Frank et al, 2003). In fleshing out why and how neighbourhood structure might affect physical activity, Frank et al (2004) divide the built environment into three basic components: transportation systems, land-use patterns and urban design characteristics. Particularly for individuals and populations in poverty, available transportation (that is, car ownership and/or public transport) may result in less frequent, slower and/or more dangerous travel (Frank et al, 2004). The availability of facilities for different types of physical activity, the physical distance and transport accessibility to facilities, the perceived quality and safety of the environment, and the natural environment (including climate) all directly play into individual participation in physical activity (Frank et al, 2004). Although the majority of the transportation/urban planning literature has not focused on health or health behaviours as outcomes, this literature is beginning to develop (Ewing et al, 2003; Frank et al, 2004).

Even after adjusting for household SES, residents from communities with higher density, greater connectivity and more land-use mix report higher rates of walking/cycling for utilitarian purposes than low-density, poorly connected and single land-use neighbourhoods (Saelens et al, 2003). Moreover, the absence of recreational and exercise facilities has been shown to increase the risk of individuals within those neighbourhoods being overweight or obese (Brownson et al, 2001; Giles-Corti and Donovan, 2003). Humpel (2002) has synthesised literature that demonstrated how factors of perceived accessibility, opportunities and aesthetic attributes of a neighbourhood environment have significant associations with physical activity.

Aside from the physical or urban design that may influence physical activity, the social environment may also play a role. For instance, neighbourhood violent crime rates have been linked to reduced physical activity (Molnar et al, 2004). Negative community perceptions (particularly of safety) appear to increase the odds of being overweight (Catlin et al, 2002) and studies have also shown that social capital and social support are protective against obesity (Cohen et al, 2006; Holtgrave and Crosby, 2006).

Neighbourhoods and obesity

Terms such as the 'obesogenicity' of environments have come to the forefront of various literatures (Swinburn, 1999). In a review of the literature on the built environment and obesity, Booth and colleagues (2005) evaluated a range of studies and although many of the studies differed in methodology, they found that, overall, greater obesity risk was associated with area of residence, resources, television, walkability, land use, sprawl and level of deprivation. Ellaway and colleagues (1997) found that material deprivation, a measure comprised as a composite of multiple factors (including car ownership, weekly household income and housing tenure), was significantly associated with higher BMI, waist circumference and prevalence of obesity. Van Lenthe and Mackenbach (2002) demonstrated similar findings in the Netherlands, where an index of material deprivation was associated with increasing mean BMI and prevalence of overweight. Cubbin and colleagues (2001) additionally found that material deprivation, measured through the Townsend Deprivation Index, was associated with cardiovascular disease risk behaviours, including physical inactivity and higher BMI.

Yet, the literature in the US that analyses obesity as an outcome is limited (Orr et al, 2003; Burdette and Whitaker, 2005; Burdette et al, 2006; Morenoff et al, 2006). A search on the PubMed database (which we conducted in July 2006) returned only two studies with the terms 'neighbourhood' and 'obesity' in the title.

Morenoff and colleagues (2006) examined how neighbourhood composition and aspects of the built environment are associated with obesity, exercise and walking, in a Chicago sample of adults. They found gender differences in the effects of mixed land use, presence of grocery/convenience stores and presence of parks and playgrounds. Two other studies have analysed obesity in children and mothers using the Fragile Families Study (Burdette and Whitaker, 2005; Burdette et al, 2006). In studies, Burdette and colleagues found that perception of one's neighbourhood as safer was associated with lower obesity prevalence among mothers (Burdette et al, 2006) and that mothers' perception of neighbourhood safety was related to higher television viewing time among their children but not to their children's outdoor play time, BMI or obesity risk (Burdette and Whitaker, 2005). However, all three of these studies were cross-sectional analyses with observational data and there are many threats to causal inference.

Some of the strongest evidence for neighbourhood effects is from a randomised policy experiment, funded by the US Department of Housing and Urban Development. 'Moving to Opportunity (MTO)' was a study and experiment that took place in five large US metropolitan areas in the mid-1990s. Very low-income families (mostly single mothers) with children under age 18 in public housing were randomised to one of three treatment groups:

(1) the experimental, or MTO, group who received housing counselling, and a Section 8 Housing Voucher that could be used to subsidise housing only if they moved to a low-poverty Census tract (<10% poverty rate);
(2) a group who received a Section 8 Housing Voucher that could be used to subsidise housing in any neighbourhood; and
(3) an in-place control group who remained eligible for public housing.

At four to seven years following randomisation to the study, researchers found significantly lower obesity prevalence among the experimental group (those randomised to move to a low-poverty neighbourhood) versus controls. The study was not designed to investigate mediators; however, the experimental group did report consuming significantly higher amounts of fruit and vegetables versus controls at follow-up, although they did not report any significantly different moderate physical activity versus controls (Orr et al, 2003). The MTO study is powerful from a methodological perspective because of its randomised design; there is very little threat to internal validity from selection bias (that is, individuals were randomised to different groups, rather than 'selecting' which group they would be in), so we are more confident in concluding that differences in neighbourhood environment – not individual characteristics – have caused the obesity differences.

Conceptual framework

Limited research has considered both the built and the sociodemographic neighbourhood simultaneously. In the case study presented in this chapter, we present a visual picture and preliminary analysis of the distribution of green space (that is, parks) and food purchasing venues in Pittsburgh in Pennsylvania and the distribution of obesity. In Figure 3.1, we present the conceptual framework guiding our interest in this area. As illustrated in this framework, neighbourhood socioeconomic characteristics, the 'food environment' and the 'physical activity environment' all contribute to the development of obesity. Thus, in this chapter, we aim to present a preliminary picture of the role of upstream social determinants and their influence on individual health-related behaviours using Pittsburgh as an example.

Our framework focuses on two major levels – neighbourhood and individual – that contribute to obesity. However, in the conceptual model we do not include, for example, environmental determinants on levels 'higher' than neighbourhood-level determinants (that is, state-level policies on transportation and/or recreation facilities) or genetic determinants on the individual level, although these factors may also be on the pathway. One way to explain excluding such factors from an analysis is by understanding where – conceptually – these factors might lie. If they are 'on the pathway' between those variables included in the conceptual model and analysis, then we might already be capturing their influence. Thus, the 'social' and 'physical' factors of interest – as presented in the figure – include neighbourhood SES and racial/ethnic composition, food purchasing venues (number and type) and green space (amount per neighbourhood). These neighbourhood factors, together, can be hypothesised to affect diet and/or physical activity through access to social and material resources (neighbourhood SES and racial composition), access to healthy and affordable food as well as a 'spatial' environment conducive to physical activity. We analyse neighbourhood sociodemographic characteristics as proxies for neighbourhood quality.

When thinking about the variables as defined in Figure 3.1, it is important to consider what each of these might capture in terms of the social and built environment. Additionally, we know that neighbourhood socioeconomic status (SES) is a valuable indication of the general economic well-being (that is, services, amenities and possibly even aesthetic value) of the neighbourhood environment. Still, other factors could be related – yet distinct. For example, racial/ethnic

Figure 3.1: Environmental determinants of diet and physical activity in relation to obesity

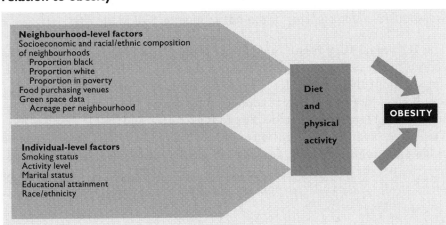

segregation is often highly correlated with neighbourhood SES. Yet there could be something specific about how racial segregation operates in the US, which contributes to diet and physical activity (and ultimately obesity), differently and distinctly from economic segregation effects on obesity. We posit that physical characteristics of the neighbourhoods, including food purchasing venues and green space, have a tangible relationship with diet and physical activity, as individuals may be geographically influenced by the options around them, in terms of making dietary and/or exercise choices.

With this understanding of 'social' factors at both individual and neighbourhood levels, we now turn to a description of these variables within one city, Pittsburgh.

Understanding place and health through an example: Pittsburgh, Pennsylvania

The City of Pittsburgh, located in southwestern Pennsylvania, is composed of 334,563 people, 67.0% non-Hispanic white, 27.8% non-Hispanic black, 3.0% Asian and 1.3% Hispanic (Lewis Mumford Center for Comparative Urban and Regional Research, 2001). With the collapse of the steel industry in the 1970s and 1980s, Pittsburgh experienced an economic decline similar to many postindustrial communities. However, the region is characterised by a stable population and a high degree of community cohesion within its neighbourhoods. Like most urban areas in the US, the spatial separation of population groups along racial/ethnic and socioeconomic lines is a central feature of the city, as discussed earlier and is a legacy, as in many other US cities, of urban renewal projects. These policies aimed to 'improve neighbourhoods' but instead disrupted well-established, close-knit communities (Fullilove, 2004). Pittsburgh's social and political history, arranged largely around its neighbourhoods, also makes Pittsburgh an ideal setting to examine neighbourhood sociodemographic factors and their relationship to obesity prevalence.

Individual-level data: looking at the distribution of BMI in the city

The Behavioral Risk Factor Surveillance System (BRFSS) is one system that collects health data from individuals across the US. The BRFSS functions with support from the Centers for Disease Control and Prevention (CDC) as a telephone health survey system conducted by the 50 state health departments, and those in District of Columbia, Puerto Rico, Guam and the US Virgin Islands. The survey includes questions on health behaviours and risk factors such as alcohol use, cancer screening, diet, physical activity, tobacco use, asthma, diabetes, hypertension, height, weight and healthcare access (CDC, 2006). The BRFSS in Allegheny County, which encompasses Pittsburgh, surveyed 1,335 adults, with a cooperation rate of 52.9%.

Each individual who participated in the BRFSS was geocoded (or linked) to a municipal neighbourhood, based on what they identified as 'their neighbourhood of residence' when asked an open-ended question on this. Our operationalisation of neighbourhood was those municipally defined in the City of Pittsburgh that have locally familiar names and spatial boundaries to Pittsburgh residents. Importantly, these municipally defined neighbourhoods share boundaries that are aggregations of, on average, between one and three US Census tracts. In our sample, the distribution of individuals per neighbourhood ranged from two individuals per neighbourhood to 72 individuals per neighbourhood. All neighbourhoods with five or fewer individuals were excluded from our analyses (n=29 individuals, n=8 neighbourhoods). Thus, the total number of neighbourhoods in our analyses was 57 and the total number of individuals was 1,251.

Body Mass Index was used to proxy obesity and was calculated as the individual's weight in kilograms divided by the square of their height measured in metres (kg/m^2). Categories of BMI followed CDC guidelines, and were defined as 'normal' (18.5–24.9), 'overweight' (25–29.9) and 'obese' (30 or greater). Individuals with BMIs under 18.5 were excluded from the analysis. We aggregated data to the neighbourhood level in order to calculate the mean BMI for each neighbourhood based on survey respondents.

Neighbourhood-level data: sociodemographics, food purchasing venues and green space

At the neighbourhood level, we were interested in looking at (1) socioeconomic and racial/ethnic composition of neighbourhoods, (2) food purchasing venues and (3) the proportion of residential green space. Socioeconomic and racial/ethnic composition data were extracted from the US Census data. We obtained information on the Census 2000 tract-level proportion of the population under the federal poverty line, median household income and median value of owner-occupied homes. We operationalised neighbourhood-level residential segregation by race/ethnicity with proportions of the tract total population who were non-Hispanic black and, separately, non-Hispanic white. Data on food purchasing venues in Pittsburgh were collected from the ReferenceUSA database, which contains detailed information on businesses in metropolitan areas across the US. Codes correspond to the following food store categories: grocery stores; convenience stores; fast-food places; carry out, pizza and sandwiches; limited-service branch restaurants; limited-service single location restaurants; specialty food stores; candy and confectionery; and coffee shops. The City of Pittsburgh Department of City Planning provided data on all of the green space, or park space, per neighbourhood. We derived the proportion of green space per neighbourhood by computing the total amount of green space in the neighbourhood, divided by the total area of the neighbourhood (in acres).

Mapping neighbourhoods and health

Our sample consisted of 1,251 individuals residing in 58 neighbourhoods. Of the 58 municipally defined neighbourhoods included in our analysis, there were 41 neighbourhoods where 50% or more of the individuals interviewed for the BRFSS were overweight or obese, 14 neighbourhoods where 75% or more of the individuals interviewed for the BRFSS were overweight or obese and three neighbourhoods where 50% or more of the individuals interviewed for the BRFSS were obese. Across all neighbourhoods, 24.2% of individuals surveyed were obese, 34.3% were overweight and 41.5% were of normal weight.

The average Pittsburgh neighbourhood (median) was 8% non-Hispanic black, with a range of 0–98%. The average Pittsburgh neighbourhood (median) was 77% non-Hispanic white, with a range of 0–99%. The average neighbourhood had 15% of its population in poverty, with a range of 0–70%.

The average Pittsburgh neighbourhood had 4% of green space, which, depending on the size of the neighbourhood, ranged from 11 to 61 acres. Neighbourhood proportion of green space ranged from 0% to 51% (0–684 acres). There were a total of 183 parks of varied acreage within the City of Pittsburgh.

In our sample, there were 1,086 food purchasing venues located within the city boundaries, the majority of which were categorised as 'limited-service restaurants'. The neighbourhood with the greatest number of venues was the 'central business district' of Pittsburgh, which is the central city or downtown area, also lower in residential accommodation. However, the neighbourhoods that followed included the four most affluent neighbourhoods (highest median neighbourhood income) of the city. Among the collection of neighbourhoods with more food purchasing venues than other neighbourhoods (that is, greater than 25 venues) were the neighbourhoods that housed two major academic institutions (Carnegie Mellon University and the University of Pittsburgh) as well as two neighbourhoods where active 'development' has been happening (that is, gentrification). When we mapped all food venues in Allegheny County (which included Pittsburgh and neighbouring cities), we saw food purchasing venues that were just outside of city boundaries. Therefore, in the case of food purchasing venues, for example, a more beneficial way to analyse this data – instead of using city boundaries – may be by forming 'buffered areas' of relevance. Map 3.1 visually illustrates the distribution of poverty at the neighbourhood level and location of food establishments.

BMI maps

In studying BMI, we depicted the normal weight/overweight/obesity categories as dots of increasing size, where the smallest dots correspond to a mean BMI falling within normal weight categories, and the largest dots correspond to a mean BMI over 30, or that the mean BMI is classified as obese. The intermediate category corresponds to a mean BMI of 25-30. Neighbourhoods without dots had less than five observations in our BRFSS sample. The obesity categories correspond

Map 3.1: Pittsburgh: proportion of the population in poverty and types of food purchasing venues

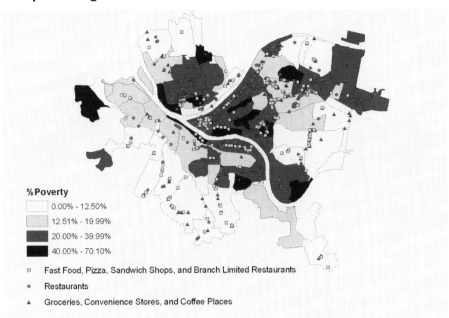

%Poverty

0.00% - 12.50%

12.51% - 19.99%

20.00% - 39.99%

40.00% - 70.10%

▫ Fast Food, Pizza, Sandwich Shops, and Branch Limited Restaurants

◆ Restaurants

▲ Groceries, Convenience Stores, and Coffee Places

Source: ReferenceUSA; US Census 2000

to the mean BMI of the neighbourhood sample (from BRFSS data). Maps 3.2 to 3.4 display the neighbourhood obesity rate juxtaposed with another variable. For Maps 3.2 and 3.3, darker-shaded neighbourhoods indicate higher proportions of people in poverty and black people (respectively), and for Map 3.4, darker-shaded neighbourhoods indicate higher proportions of green space.

Map 3.2 illustrates that we observed higher mean BMI in more impoverished neighbourhoods, but we observe that there are also some high-poverty neighbourhoods with low BMI. The map illustrates that regardless of poverty status, few neighbourhoods (n=10) have BMI in the 'normal' range (19.1–24.9). Map 3.3 shows that black people are clustered in parts of the city, similar to Map 3.2, that have lower income. Map 3.3 also illustrates higher BMI in neighbourhoods with a higher percentage of black residents. Map 3.4 visually depicts the relationship between the proportion of green space per neighbourhood and mean BMI. Larger dots, representing higher mean BMI, are more concentrated in lighter-shaded neighbourhoods, or those neighbourhoods with lesser proportions of green space.

Map 3.2: Pittsburgh: distribution of BMI and the proportion of people in poverty per neighbourhood

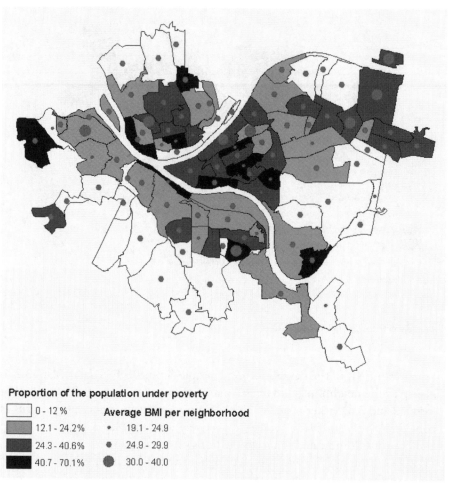

Proportion of the population under poverty

0 - 12 %	**Average BMI per neighborhood**
12.1 - 24.2%	• 19.1 - 24.9
24.3 - 40.6%	• 24.9 - 29.9
40.7 - 70.1%	● 30.0 - 40.0

Source: US Census Bureau (2006); the Allegheny County BRFSS

Map 3.3: Pittsburgh: distribution of BMI and the proportion of black people per neighbourhood

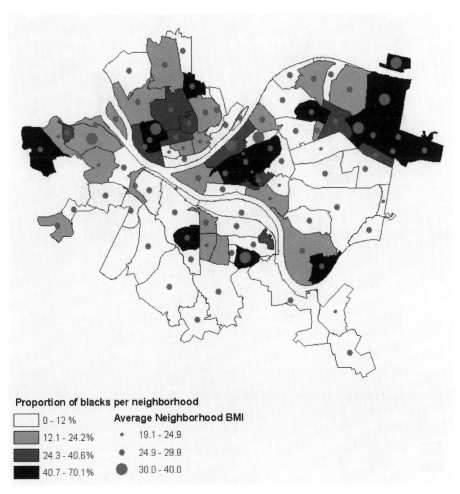

Proportion of blacks per neighborhood

☐	0 - 12 %
▨	12.1 - 24.2%
▨	24.3 - 40.6%
■	40.7 - 70.1%

Average Neighborhood BMI

- · 19.1 - 24.9
- • 24.9 - 29.9
- ● 30.0 - 40.0

Source: US Census Bureau (2006); the Allegheny County BRFSS

Map 3.4: Pittsburgh: distribution of BMI and the proportion of green space per neighbourhood

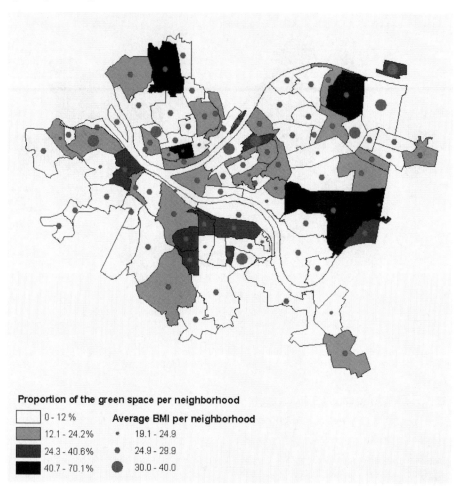

Proportion of the green space per neighborhood

	0 - 12 %	**Average BMI per neighborhood**
	12.1 - 24.2%	• 19.1 - 24.9
	24.3 - 40.6%	• 24.9 - 29.9
	40.7 - 70.1%	● 30.0 - 40.0

Source: City of Pittsburgh Department of City Planning

Discussion

The objectives of this chapter were to discuss how residential neighbourhood environments and obesity are connected, or more broadly speaking, the relationship between 'place' and 'health'. Our interests developed from seeking to understand how the residential environments could influence health behaviours related to obesity, such as diet and physical activity. Pittsburgh was an ideal setting for a case study in that the data on both individuals (BMI data) and neighbourhoods (socioeconomic and built environment data) were available. The issue of data availability is often an obstacle to the execution of work in this field.

One challenge with regard to the neighbourhoods and health research agenda is the issue of boundaries: How should neighbourhoods be defined conceptually, and what are the resulting empirical problems with estimation should these boundaries be inaccurate? What are the boundaries that correspond to food shopping or physical activity practices? The bounding or definition of neighbourhoods in neighbourhood health research has garnered a lot of attention, as a topic of contention (O'Campo, 2005). Residents rarely conceive of neighbourhoods along Census block or Census tract boundaries (O'Campo, 2005), although this is the unit of data that is often available and utilised in health studies (Kawachi and Berkman, 2003). How an outsider defines neighbourhood boundaries might be different from how a resident him/herself does, and there is likely to be considerable variability within a certain neighbourhood about defining that neighbourhood. Moreover, boundaries of neighbourhoods may not be fixed for any one person or population, but may be reliant on specific purposes, processes or health outcomes (Diez Roux, 2004; Diez Roux and Aiello, 2005; O'Campo, 2005).

Additional challenges include identification of the specific characteristics and neighbourhood exposures that are culturally relevant and valid to the community of interest. While a challenge for most 'neighbourhood effects' research, it is also such for most observational studies in general; selection is a threat to validity for causal inference – for example, individuals do not randomly select which neighbourhood to reside in, and the characteristics they use to choose a neighbourhood are often strongly associated with health (Diez Roux, 2004). Selection is the main threat to validity for causal inference in our study; we cannot deduce that neighbourhood factors are causal.

Neighbourhoods may exhibit different effects for different groups of people. There may be differences in the way in which groups of people interact with their neighbourhood environment according to race/ethnicity, gender and age. For example, in prior research with immigrant and non-immigrant low-income women, Dubowitz and colleagues (2005) found that immigrant women were more willing to travel long distances for their food purchasing (and thus their diet was less affected by the constraints of what was proximally available to them).

Yet despite the challenges doing research with respect to neighbourhood effects, there is a tremendous amount that we have yet to learn about the social context and covariation of inequality and health. Many of the descriptive patterns and mechanisms by which neighbourhood effects manifest into health outcomes are an important aspect of the research, and yet are under-explored. Thus, asking why we observe such selection and sorting of individuals into different neighbourhoods, why it is that social position is so linked to neighbourhood quality, are questions directly related to health and health disparities. Much of the research on neighbourhood and health has focused on quality of neighbourhood, operationalised through Census measures of SES, not material or social aspects of neighbourhoods. In this way, Census measures are proxies for material or social dimensions of neighbourhoods that affect health. Thus, there is great potential for additional neighbourhood and health research that incorporates specific physical, material or social aspects of neighbourhoods that matter for health. In our case study of Pittsburgh, we observed an initial picture of how the physical (specifically green/park space and food purchasing venues) and sociodemographic (poverty and racial composition) environment of neighbourhoods may be related to obesity.

Although our research extends the extant literature on the built environment and diet and physical activity, our study is limited by our measures of built environment. For example, we were unable to capture resources in addition to those of green space and food purchasing venues, such as community and social services and crime rates that also contribute to influencing the neighbourhood environment and subsequently physical activity and potentially diet. There may additionally be a 'neighbourhood psychosocial context' that influences health behaviours. Social contagion models suggest that people's behaviour is influenced by the norms or values of those around them (Jencks and Mayer, 1990; Crane, 1991). Therefore, cultural norms and/or exposure to chronic stressors (Ross, 2000) could directly contribute to health behaviours.

Researchers have also examined how urban design characteristics influence choice. For example, when making decisions around transportation to and from destinations, distance, accessibility, proximity of multiple destinations in addition to safety are just some of the factors that individuals might consider. Thus, the width of streets and pavements, the location of pedestrian crossings, and the landscape all affect an individual's perception of neighbourhood environments.

Our analysis of features and individuals of Pittsburgh demonstrates spatial patterning in obesity that may be associated with social context and physical patterning of resources. Importantly, it merges public health research with urban planning and development. Researchers and policy makers have long been aware of the need for transdisciplinary action, particularly within the area of urban health. However, the reality of bridging fields together is often difficult. Yet, for the case of obesity, when we understand that 24% of US adults were overweight in 1960, 47% were overweight in 1980 and 64% were obese in 2000, we are obliged to better understand and more thoroughly examine what it is about our environment, both the physical and socioeconomic aspects of our neighbourhoods, that has changed. With this insight, we are much better equipped to tackle the public's health.

References

Acevedo-Garcia, D., Lochner, K.A., Osypuk, T.L. and Subramanian, S.V. (2003) 'Future directions in residential segregation and health research: a multilevel approach,' *American Journal of Public Health* 93: 215-21.

Berkman, L. and Kawachi, I. (2000) *Social epidemiology*, New York: Oxford University Press.

Block, J.P., Scribner, R.A. and DeSalvo, K.B. (2004) 'Fast food, race/ethnicity, and income: A geographic analysis', *American Journal of Preventative Medicine* 27(3): 211-17.

Booth, K.M., Pinkston, M.M. and Poston, W.S. (2005) 'Obesity and the built environment', *Journal of the American Dietetic Association* 105(5): 110-17.

Brownell, K.D (2005) 'Does a 'toxic' environment make obesity inevitable?', *Obesity Management* 1(2): 52-5.

Brownson, R.C., Baker, E.A., Housemann, R.A., Brennan, L.K. and Bacak, S.J. (2001) 'Environmental and policy determinants of physical activity in the United States', *American Journal of Public Health* 91: 1995-2003.

Burdette, H.L. and Whitaker, R.C. (2005) 'A national study of neighborhood safety, outdoor play, television viewing, and obesity in preschool children', *Pediatrics* 116: 657-62.

Burdette, H.L., Wadden, T.A. and Whitaker, R.C. (2006) 'Neighborhood safety, collective efficacy, and obesity in women with young children', *Obesity* 14: 518-25.

Catlin, T.K., Simoes, E.J. and Brownson, R.C. (2002) 'Brownson environmental and policy factors associated with overweight among adults in Missouri', *American Journal of Health Promotion* 17(4): 249-58.

CDC (Centers for Disease Control and Prevention) (2006) 'Behavioral risk factor surveillance site homepage', www.cdc.gov/brfss/ (retrieved 15 September 2006).

Chang, V. and Lauderdale, D. (2005) 'Income disparities in Body Mass Index and obesity in the United States: 1971–2002', *Archives of Internal Medicine* 165(18): 2122-28.

Chang, V.W. (2006) 'Racial residential segregation and weight status among U.S. adults', *Social Science and Medicine* 63(5): 1289-303.

Cohen, D., Finch, B., Bower, A. and Sastry, N. (2006) 'Collective efficacy and obesity: the potential influence of social factors on health', *Social Science and Medicine* 62(3): 769-78.

Collins, C. and Williams, D.R. (2001) 'Racial residential segregation: a fundamental cause of racial disparities in health', *Public Health Reports* 116: 404-16.

Crane, J. (1991) 'The epidemic theory of ghettos and neighborhood effects on dropping out and teenage childbearing', *American Journal of Sociology* 96: 1236-59.

Cubbin, C., Hadden, W.C. and Winkleby, M. A. (2001) 'Neighborhood context and cardiovascular disease risk factors: the contribution of material deprivation', *Ethnicity and Disease* 11: 687-700.

Denney, J.T., Krueger, P.M., Rogers, R.G. and Boardman, J. (2004) 'Race/ethnic and sex differentials in body mass among US adults', *Ethnicity and Disease* 14(3): 389-98.

Diez Roux, A. (2004) 'Estimating neighborhood health effects: the challenges of causal inference in a complex world', *Journal of Social Science and Medicine* 58(10): 1953-60.

Diez Roux, A.V. and Aiello, A.E. (2005) 'Multi-level analysis of infectious diseases', *Journal of Infectious Diseases* 191(Suppl 1): S25-S33.

Diez Roux, A.V., Nieto F.J. and Caulfield, L. et al (1999) 'Neighborhood differences in diet: the atherosclerosis risk in communities (aric) study', *Journal of Epidemiology and Community Health* 53: 55-63.

Drewnowski, A. and Specter, S.E. (2004) 'Poverty and obesity: the role of energy density and energy costs', *American Journal of Clinical Nutrition* 79: 6-16.

Dubowitz, T., Acevedo-Garcia, D., Salkeld, J., Lindsay, A.C., Subramanian, S.V. and Peterson, K.E. (2005) 'Lifecourse, immigrant status and acculturation in food purchasing and preparation among low-income mothers', *Public Health and Nutrition* 10(4): 395-404.

Ellaway, A., Anderson, A. and Macintyre, S. (1997) 'Does area of residence affect body size and shape?' *International Journal of Obesity and Related Metabolic Disorders* 21: 304-8.

Ewing, R., Schmid, T.L., Killingsworth, R., Zlot, A. and Raudenbush, S. (2003) 'Relationship between urban sprawl and physical activity, obesity, and morbidity', *American Journal of Health Promotion* 18: 47-57.

Flegal, K.M., Carroll, M., Ogden, C. and Johnson, C. (2002) 'Prevalence and trends in obesity among US adults: 1999–2000', *Journal of American Medical Association* 288(14): 1723-7.

Frank, L.D., Engelke, P.O. and Schmid, T.L. (2003) *Health and community design: the impact of the built environment on physical activity*, Washington, DC: Island Press,.

Frank, L.D., Andresen, M.A. and Schmid, T.L. (2004) 'Obesity relationships with community design, physical activity, and time spent in cars', *American Journal of Preventative Medicine* 27(2): 87-96.

Fullilove, M. (2004) *Root shock: How tearing up city neighborhoods hurts America and what we can do about it*, New York, NY: Ballantine/One World.

Giles-Corti, B. and Donovan, R.J. (2003) 'Relative influences of individual, social environmental, and physical environmental correlates of walking', *American Journal of Public Health* 93: 1583-9.

Hedley, A., Ogden, C., Johnson, C., Carroll, M., Curtin, L. and Flegal, K. (2004) 'Prevalence of overweight and obesity among US children, adolescents, and adults: 1999-2002', *Journal of the American Medical Association* 291: 2847-50.

Holtgrave, D. and Crosby, R. (2006) 'Is social capital a protective factor against obesity and diabetes? Findings from an exploratory study', *Annals of Epidemiology* 16(5): 406-8.

Humpel, N. (2002) 'Environmental factors associated with adults' participation in physical activity: a review', *American Journal of Preventative Medicine* 22(3): 188-99.

Iceland, J., Sharpe, C. and Steinmetz, E. (2005) 'Class differences in African American residential patterns in U.S. metropolitan areas: 1990–2000', *Social Science Research* 34(1): 252-66.

Jencks, C. and Mayer, S.E. (1990) 'The social consequences of growing up in a poor neighborhood', in L.E. Lynn and M.G.H. McGeary (eds) *Inner city poverty in the United States*, Washington, DC: National Academy Press: 111-86.

Kawachi, I. and Berkman, L.F. (2003) *Introduction: Neighborhoods and health.* Oxford, NY: Oxford University Press: 1-19.

Lewis Mumford Center for Comparative Urban and Regional Research (2001) *Segregation: Whole population, Census 2000 Data*, Albany, NY; State University of New York at Albany.

Massey, D.S. (1995) 'Getting away with murder: segregation and violent crime in urban America', *University of Pennsylvania Law Review* 143: 1203-32.

McTigue, K.M., Garrett, J.M. and Popkin, B.M. (2002) 'Are young overweight adults destined for obesity?', *Clinician Reviews* 12(9): 29.

Molnar, B.E., Gortmaker, S.L., Bull, F.C. and Buka, S.L. (2004) '"Unsafe to play?" neighborhood disorder and lack of safety predict reduced physical activity among urban children and adolescents', *American Journal of Health Promotion* 18(5): 378-86.

Moore, L.V. and Diez Roux, A.V. (2006) 'Associations of neighborhood characteristics with location and type of food stores', *American Journal of Public Health* 96: 325-31.

Morenoff, J.D., Diez Roux, A.V., Osypuk, T. and Hansen, B. (2006) 'Residential environments and obesity: what can we learn about policy interventions from observational studies?', in National Poverty Center, *Health Effects of Non-Health Policy,* Bethesda, MD: National Poverty Center, University of Michigan.

Morland, K., Wing, S. and Diez Roux, A. (2002) 'The contextual effect of the local food environment on residents' diets: the atherosclerosis risks in communities study', *American Journal of Public Health* 92: 6.

O'Campo, P. (2005) 'Multilevel modeling in perinatal research', http://128.249.232.90/archives/cdc/mchepi/february2005/ mchepifebruary2005transcript.pdf; www.uic.edu/sph/cade/mchepi/meetings/ feb2005/index.htm (retrieved 4 June 2006).

Orr, L., Feins, J.D., Jacob, R., Beecroft, E., Sanbonmatsu, L., Katz, L.F., Liebman, J.F. and Kling, J.R. (2003) *Moving to opportunity interim impacts evaluation*, Washington, DC: US Department of Housing and Urban Development Office of Policy Development and Research.

Poortinga, W. (2006) 'Social relations or social capital? Individual and community health effects of bonding social capital', *Social Science and Medicine* 63(1): 255-70.

Popkin, B.M. (1998) 'The nutrition transition and its health implication in lower income countries', *Public Health Nutrition* 1: 5-21.

Popkin, B.M. (2003) 'The nutrition transition in the developing world', *Developing Policy Review* 21: 581-97.

ReferenceUSA database. Accessed at www.referenceusa.com and the Carnegie Library of Pittsburgh, Pennsylvania.

Ross, C.E. (2000) 'Walking, exercising, and smoking: does neighborhood matter?' *Social Science and Medicine* 5: 265-74.

Saelens, B.E., Sallis, J.F. and Frank, L.D. (2003) 'Environmental correlates of walking and cycling: the finding from the transportation, urban design, and planning literatures', *Annals of Behavioral Medicine* 25: 80-91.

Sampson, R.J., Raudenbush, S.W. and Earls, F. (1997) 'Neighborhoods and violent crime: a multilevel study of collective efficacy', *Science* 277(5328): 918-24.

Schoenborn, C.A., Adams, P.F. and Barnes, P.M. (2002) *Body weight status of adults: United States, 1997–98. Advance data from vital and health statistics*, Hyattsville, MD: National Center for Health Statistics.

Schulz, A.J., Williams, D.R., Israel, B.A. and Bex Lempert, L. (2002) 'Racial and spatial relations as fundamental determinants of health in Detroit', *Milbank Quarterly* 80(4): 677.

Shohaimi, S., Welch, A., Bingham, S., Luben, R., Day, N., Wareham, N. and Khaw, K.T. (2004) 'Residential area deprivation predicts fruit and vegetable consumption independently of individual educational level and occupational social class: a cross-sectional population study in the Norfolk cohort of the European prospective investigation into cancer', *Journal of Epidemiology and Community Health* 58(8): 686-91.

Sobal, J. and Stunkard, A.J. (1989) 'Socioeconomic status and obesity: a review of the literature', *Psychology Bulletin* 105: 260-75.

Stunkard, A.J. (1996) 'Socioeconomic status and obesity', *Ciba Foundation Symposium* 201: 174-93.

Swinburn, B. (1999) 'Dissecting obesogenic environments: the development and application of a framework for identifying and prioritizing environmental interventions for obesity', *Preventive Medicine* 29(6): 563.

US Census Bureau (2006) 'North American industry classification system homepage', www.census.gov/epcd/www/naicsdev.htm (retrieved 15 September 2006).

Van Lenthe, F.J. and Mackenbach, J.P. (2002) 'Neighbourhood deprivation and overweight: the GLOBE study', *International Journal of Obesity and Related Metabolic Disorders* 26: 234-40.

Zenk, S.N., Schulz, A.J., Israel, B.A., James, S.A., Bao, S. and Mark, L. (2005) 'Neighborhood racial composition, neighborhood poverty, and the spatial accessibility of supermarkets in metropolitan Detroit', *American Journal of Public Health* 95(4): 660-7.

FOUR

Reinventing healthy and sustainable communities: reconnecting public health and urban planning

Mary E. Northridge, Elliott D. Sclar, Annie Feighery, Maryann Z. Fiebach and Emily Karpel Kurtz

Introduction

The world has an unprecedented opportunity to improve the health and lives of billions of people by adopting practical approaches to meeting the United Nations (UN) Millennium Development Goals. The Task Force on Improving the Lives of Slum Dwellers has identified strategies for managing a projected near doubling of the urban population over the next three decades. We contend that this challenge can be met if local authorities and national governments work closely with the urban poor through open and participatory processes that give them a voice in decisions about the infrastructure and public services that affect their lives. Building on earlier work that aims to reconnect public health and urban planning, we identify four core themes that we consider as transferable best principles, which will be essential in bringing policies and programmes up to scale to meet the 21st-century health challenge of slums and cities: interdisciplinary engagement, gender equality, sustainable development and democratic institution building. By developing policies and programmes that are pro-poor, the health and lives of all of us stand to improve. Indeed, our best hope for reinventing healthy and sustainable communities is to place the urban poor at the very centre of policy formation and investment processes. In this way, the outcomes – healthy populations and sustainable communities – will take care of themselves.

Interdisciplinary scholarship and training

This chapter is written in tribute to our students at Columbia University, and by extension, to all past, current and future students who are committed to answering societies' big questions (for example, 'Will the poor always be with us?' – see Darity, 2003) and solving the world's big problems (for example, achieving the UN Millennium Development Goals). Our ideas have been incubated in the course entitled 'Interdisciplinary Planning for Health' that two of us (Mary E. Northridge and Elliott D. Sclar) have co-taught over the past nine years and enhanced by the contributions of successive waves of students. Indeed, the three other co-authors were all former students on this course and conducted apt research used in conceiving our ideas and birthing this chapter (Emily Karpel Kurtz in 2004, Maryann Z. Fiebach in 2005 and Annie Feighery in 2006).

The case study in future urban transport presented here is part of an ongoing research and training project at the Center for Sustainable Urban Development at Columbia University founded by Professor Sclar. Parts of the presentation were derived from an Urban Planning Program studio conducted in collaboration with colleagues at the Mailman School of Public Health and the University of Nairobi. Here we expand on core concepts and adapt an ecological model we had previously developed (Northridge et al, 2003; Schulz and Northridge, 2004) to make more explicit the connections between societal, community and interpersonal determinants of population health and well-being for the inhabitants of the Ruiru municipality of Nairobi, Kenya.

Overarching goal and specific aims of this task

Our hope for this chapter is to bolster our thinking on the pathways through which societal inequalities affect population health and well-being, with a particular focus on meeting the 21st-century health challenge of slums and cities (Sclar et al, 200b). We begin with an overview of the scope and scale of global poverty and give due emphasis to the growing urban crisis of slums (Garau et al, 2005). Next, we argue that the fields of public health and urban planning need to return to their entwined roots in the reform efforts of the 19th-century industrialised cities (Sclar and Northridge, 2001) in order to be effective in meeting the contemporary challenge of slums (Northridge et al, 2003). Then, we hone in on four core themes (interdisciplinary engagement, gender equality, sustainable development and democratic institution building) that we dub transferable best principles, as they can potentially be applied across programmes and policies to make enduring contributions to the important challenges resulting from the current wave of global urbanisation (Sclar et al, 2005b). Subsequently, we present a case study of the Ruiru municipality within the larger metropolitan area of Nairobi, Kenya, in rethinking joint public health and urban planning solutions to future urban transport needs (Sclar and Touber, 2006). We end the chapter with an exhortation to embrace what we believe is the only realistic strategy for reinventing healthy and sustainable communities, namely, placing the urban poor at the very centre of their policy formulation and investment processes.

Re-imagining a more equitable world

The Millennium Development Goals

At the Millennium Summit in September 2000, the states of the UN reaffirmed their commitment to working towards a more equitable world through a new global partnership to reduce extreme poverty. Eight Millennium Development Goals (MDGs) grew out of the agreements and resolutions. The MDGs have since become the basis of a global effort led by former UN Secretary General Kofi Annan to address global poverty, including the extensive environmental degradation and health problems of slums (that is, precarious housing submarkets – see Sclar and Northridge, 2003) and slum dwellers (now numbering more than a billion of the world's poorest urban residents). To provide planning and policy substance to this effort, the Millennium Development Project was organised to advise the UN on how to implement the MDGs. To facilitate this work, the challenges of the eight MDGs were assigned to 10 task forces consisting of outside experts, UN specialists and representatives of relevant international organisations.

Task Force 8, the Task Force on Improving the Lives of Slum Dwellers, was specifically charged with target 11 of the MDGs: 'Have achieved by 2020 a significant improvement in the lives of at least 100 million slum dwellers'. The Task Force 8 members have since proposed the following reformulation of target 11: 'By 2020, improving substantially the lives of at least 100 million slum dwellers, while providing adequate alternatives to slum formation' (Garau et al, 2005, p 3).

The urban crisis

The fastest-growing proportion of the global population is the urban population in the poorest countries of the world (Northridge and Sclar, 2003). According to UN estimates (UN Population Division, 1999), while the global population over the next 30 years is expected to increase at an annual rate of less than 1% per year (that is, 0.97%), the urbanised population of the less-developed regions of the world will increase by almost 3% per year (that is, 2.67%). The implications of this impending urban crisis are staggering. Presently, there are almost two billion people living in urbanised regions of the developing world, nearly one billion of whom face problems of wrenching poverty, malnutrition, inadequate or no housing, poor quality of or a severe lack of drinking water, inadequate waste disposal systems and drainage, and other harsh physical and social conditions of day-to-day life that contribute to high rates of premature mortality, infectious diseases such as tuberculosis, malaria and HIV/AIDS, injuries and domestic violence, depression and anxiety, poor maternal and child health outcomes and many other grave public health concerns (Garau et al, 2005).

By 2030, it is expected that the current two billion city dwellers will double to approximately four billion in a global population that, by then, will total close to eight billion. The number of cities with more than five million inhabitants (termed 'megacities') will grow from 41 at present to an expected 59 by 2015. Most of these megacities will be located in the least-developed parts of the world; indeed, only 10 of the current 41 megacities are located in developed countries, and only one of the expected 18 new megacities will be located in a developed country. Geographically, cities of all sizes are growing fastest in the poorest regions of the world, especially in Africa and Latin America, where urbanisation is being spurred by civil wars, natural disasters and plummeting agricultural prices (Northridge and Sclar, 2002). Thus, the sheer number of people living in cities in general, and in urban poverty in particular, demands focused attention on the connections between what is planned and built and the health and well-being of the people who live there.

Slums and slum dwellers

While their physical forms vary by place and over time, slums are uniformly characterised by inadequate provision of basic infrastructure and public services necessary to sustain life and health, such as access to adequate clean water, sanitation facilities and drainage (Garau et al, 2005). Buildings made of flimsy materials are prone to ignite, frequently collapse and offer scant protection against the elements, leaving their residents vulnerable to injury, violence, illness and death (Sclar and Northridge, 2003). Further, since many of these settlements are illegal, slum dwellers are excluded from many of the attributes of urban life that are critical to full citizenship but that remain a monopoly of a privileged minority: political voice, secure and good-quality housing, safety and the rule of law, good education, affordable health services, decent transport, adequate incomes and access to economic vitality and credit (Garau et al, 2005).

According to Task Force 8 members, if the urban context of poverty is not directly addressed, it will be impossible to achieve the MDGs (Garau et al, 2005). In their words:

> What is needed is the vision, the commitment, and the resources to bring all actors together and do the sensible things that are the tasks of well governed cities – providing political and economic opportunity, improving services and the quality of public space, planning for future needs, expanding local sources of revenue, attracting investment – in active cooperation and dialogue with all citizens, especially slum dwellers, both women and men. (Garau et al, 2005, pp 2-3)

We believe that the mandate of Task Force 8 might be meaningfully advanced with more explicit attention to the pathways whereby improved urban planning might lead to better population health and well-being for slum dwellers, and thereby a healthier and more equitable world for all.

Reconnecting public health and urban planning

Value added of unity in thought and action

Six years ago, we first articulated a joint urban planning and public health framework for use in assessing the health impacts of proposed projects, policies and programmes within and across population groups (Northridge and Sclar, 2003).

Since then, we have set about trying to better explicate our conceptual models using, for example, housing and health interventions (Northridge et al, 2003), environmental health promotion (Schulz and Northridge, 2004) and childhood asthma (Spielman et al, 2006) as case studies. All of our joint public health and urban planning conceptual models published to date have been US-based, and none has explicitly focused on gender inequalities.

Over the past decade especially, others in both the public health and urban planning professions have likewise argued for reunification of these fields through better frameworks for thinking about how places influence health (Stephens et al, 1997; Freudenberg, 2000; Macintyre et al, 2002; Dannenberg et al, 2003; Frumkin, 2003; Kaplan and Kaplan, 2003; Srinivasan et al, 2003; Corburn, 2004; Galea and Vlahov, 2005). In the US, much of the focus has been on promoting environmental change as a means to increase physical activity (Hoehner et al, 2003; Spence and Leeb, 2003; Brownson et al, 2004; Sallis et al, 2004).

Examining the evidence

In 2005, the Transportation Research Board of the National Academies in the US published a landmark report entitled *Does the built environment influence physical activity? Examining the evidence* (TRB and Institute of Medicine of the National Academies, 2005). As part of that effort, we were asked to prepare a working paper on 'Promoting interdisciplinary curricula and training in transportation, land use, physical activity, and health' (Sclar et al, 2005b). Through that exercise, we concluded that the base of theory and scientific evidence that connects specific design configurations of the built environment to specific use patterns and exposures and ultimately to specific population health outcomes is lacking (Sclar et al, 2005b).

Nonetheless, we believe that the aggregate work completed to date is sufficiently plausible and robust in its broadest causal outlines and preliminary findings that prudence requires us to act by integrating knowledge across sectors to guide proposed projects and policies (Sclar et al, 2005b). Given the scope and scale of the global urban crisis, we recommend applying the best principles derived through experience even as we strive to further detail and rigorously test apt conceptual models through focused research and evaluated interventions (Schulz and Northridge, 2004).

Redefining core themes

What we mean by best principles

In light of the ambiguity that surrounds policy-oriented programmes in public health and urban planning, we stress here the need to develop such programmes with an emphasis on transferable core themes or best principles (Sclar et al, 2005b). We focus on best principles rather than on best practices in order to underscore the need to extract the core themes of an initiative from the context in which they are carried out. In the development of new programmes, we are often confronted with situations where the historical and cultural contexts vary greatly, even as the ostensible activities are the same. In such cases, best practices do not always transfer readily across sites. On the other hand, best principles remind us that, while local organisational settings can be critically different, the encompassed programme activities that we are seeking to understand may have underlying themes or principles that may be usefully adapted by other communities to enhance both individual and population health and well-being (Burrus et al, 2006).

The application of best principles requires us to have a critical understanding of the goals and constraints of different organisations as we develop new programmes. Put slightly differently, process will be as important as plan in creating innovative projects to effectively address the 21st-century health challenge of slums and cities (Sclar et al, 2005b). Based on a review of the relevant literature and engaged conversations among ourselves and others, we nominate four best principles – interdisciplinary engagement, gender equality, sustainable development and democratic institution building – that we believe are core to our joint public health and urban planning model, and can be useful in meeting the challenge of the MDGs.

Interdisciplinary engagement

It has been posited that in order for the academy to provide a stronger basis for achieving scientific and societal advances, it must develop programmes that are truly interdisciplinary in both form and content (Mitrany and Stokols, 2005; Sclar et al, 2005b). Interdisciplinary programmes involve a transformative experience among the involved faculty and students. In some qualitatively significant manner, interdisciplinary engagement dissolves the boundaries of the original disciplinary perspectives and contributes to the emergence of an integrative approach that is not possible through more customary forms of cooperation by experts from different fields.

Multidisciplinary, cross-disciplinary and transdisciplinary are descriptors of more commonplace situations that cut across disciplinary boundaries. In these cases, participants contribute their expertise to a particular circumscribed challenge, but they fail to change either the research questions they ask or the methods they use to investigate them in any meaningful way (Sclar et al, 2005b). Further, they do not view themselves as involved in an evolutionary process that is changing the nature of the mission in qualitative or quantitative terms. The end result of such ventures is typically a collaborative solution to a specific problem, rather than a restructuring of the research enterprise. By comparison, the type of interdisciplinary cooperation we describe can lead to institutional and structural change and can be scaled up to meet the enormous yet achievable challenges presented by the MDGs.

Nieves (2002, p 216) argues the point more eloquently:

Interdisciplinary and multidisciplinary research involve the study of a given subject from the assembled approaches of multiple disciplines (Yang, 2000). A multidisciplinary approach seeks to gain new knowledge through the combination of purely disciplinary approaches, much like a patchwork quilt. Interdisciplinary research substantially integrates traditional disciplinary approaches and is often referred to as a kind of seamless woven garment. The advantage of these approaches is the ability to combine the expertise of different disciplines through the exchange of concepts, ideas, and techniques into the development of a comprehensive framework for explanation of a social phenomenon (Yang, 2000).

Further, Nieves (2002, p 216) recognises that 'interdisciplinary research demands a mastery of many different fields that threaten the academy's norms of highly specialized scholars and yielding more truths in our understanding of the interlocking systems of oppression that have defined race, class, gender, and sexuality in American life'.

Gender equality

In singling out gender equality for explicit attention in this chapter, we in no way consider it more important than other forms of equality based on, for example, race/ethnicity, sexuality, disability, age, nationality and religion (Krieger, 2001). Rather, we seek here to directly address MDG 3 – 'Promote gender equality and empower women' – and enhance and expand understanding of gender-based MDG targets (for example, Target 4: 'Eliminate gender disparity in primary and secondary education, preferably by 2005, and in all levels of education no later than 2015') and recommendations (for example, as part of Recommendation 2: 'Focus on women's and girls' health, including reproductive health, and education outcomes, access to economic and political opportunities, right to control assets, and freedom from violence').

The crux of gender equality concerns (un)equal treatment on the basis of a socially defined construct that varies over time and place. Gender theorists in both public health and urban planning have thoughtfully articulated this concept. In her glossary for social epidemiology, Krieger (2001, p 694) asserts:

> Gender refers to a social construct regarding culture-bound conventions, roles, and behaviors for, as well as relations between and among, women and men and boys and girls. Gender roles vary across a continuum and both gender relations and biological expressions of gender vary within and across societies, typically in relation to social divisions premised on power and authority (for example, class, race/ethnicity, nationality, religion).

In the Introduction to their edited volume, *Gender and planning: A reader*, Fainstein and Servon (2005, p 3) likewise argue:

> When we study gender, we are studying a system in which women, men, gays, lesbians, and the trans-gendered are implicated and entwined. One cannot exist without the other. Gender has to do with the behaviors, expectations, and norms confronting each group *in relation to* the other.

They further explain (Fainstein and Servon, 2005, p 3):

> The temporal aspect of gender is as important as the relational one. Unlike the categories male and female, or man and woman, which are relatively static, the category of gender is dynamic. And therein lies its power. Gender has to do with socially constructed notions about appropriate roles and behaviors for men and women, but these roles change over time.

What the MDGs explicitly seek to address in calling for gender equality is *sexism*, defined by Krieger (2001, p 694) as:

> inequitable gender relationships and ... institutional and interpersonal practices whereby members of dominant groups (usually men) accrue privileges by subordinating other gender groups (typically women) and justify these practices via ideologies of innate superiority, difference, or deviance.

When gender equality and sexism are understood in these terms, the MDGs go far beyond championing women's and girls' rights. Rather, they call for institutional and societal change to protect oppressed gender groups from any restrictions against their lives through judgements or actions.

Fainstein and Servon (2005, p 6) sum up the implications of a gender perspective in the following way:

> Understanding gender as a system comprising women and men does not imply that shifting the dominant perspective means less for men. It would be wrong to think of what we envision as a zero-sum game, in which any change in one direction necessitates a loss from somewhere else. We believe that the kind of changes that would result from looking at problems through a gendered lens would function to make the pie bigger for all of us, rather than dividing up the same pie differently.

Sustainable development

While much has been written about and debated regarding sustainable development, we endorse the following succinct definition as set forth by Task Force 8 members: 'Sustainable development is that special kind of development that does not depend upon the whims of donors or on the vagaries of political fluctuations or markets, but that is anchored in a shared vision that people themselves can be drivers of good policy and action' (Garau et al, 2005, p xv). Task Force 8 members also recommended that governments and international agencies recognise the urban poor as active agents and not passive beneficiaries of development (Garau et al, 2005).

Sherry R. Arnstein (1969), in her influential urban planning article 'A ladder of citizen participation', graded levels of participation on a scale from non-participation (manipulation, therapy) through degrees of tokenism (informing, consultation, placation), up to steps of citizen power (partnership, delegated power, citizen control). She considered true citizen participation to involve a redistribution of power that enabled those who were historically excluded from political and economic processes to be deliberately included in current and future processes.

From a public health perspective, community-based participatory research has been invoked as a promising strategy for promoting civil society and helping to eliminate egregious disparities in health and healthcare for those without sufficient resources to pay high costs for safe and affordable housing, education across the lifecourse and adequate and respectful medical care (Northridge et al, 2005). The process of gaining participation of the impoverished across sites in the developed and developing world will no doubt differ, but without the active involvement of those affected by development policies and programmes, they stand no hope of being sustained.

To summarise, it is strictly impossible to separate the outcomes of sustainable development from the processes through which they are achieved. Indeed, in truly participatory processes, the outcomes take care of themselves. For well-informed participation to occur, transparency is necessary, but not sufficient. It requires a fundamental redefinition of the political relationship between government and all citizens, particularly the urban poor (Garau et al, 2005).

Democratic institution building

The last core theme or best principle that we identify here is that of democratic institution building. Task Force 8 members have reviewed ample evidence over the past 20 years, which has demonstrated that the urban poor themselves can provide the central impetus for change towards good governance (Garau et al, 2005). They further assert that:

> Governments, especially local governments, have also demonstrated that they can develop the capacity to use their mandates and resources for sound and participatory urban development policy, if such policies are rooted in a political leadership that is committed to a democratic and equitable vision of civil society in all spheres of government. (Garau et al, 2005, p 2)

Policies are never neutral. Neither are institutions. We advocate supporting and enacting pro-poor policies and changing institutions as needed to ensure that they are accountable to the urban poor. The challenge of the MDGs can be met if local authorities and national governments work closely with urban populations and their associations through open and participatory processes.

International agencies have also embraced this strategy. According to Task Force 8 members (Garau et al, 2005, p 85):

> In the mid-1990s, the integration of poverty alleviation became a more central component of lending strategies. The introduction of more flexible lending instruments facilitated the development of a new generation of interventions combining macroeconomic stabilization, national sectoral policies, and integrated programs to alleviate poverty and improve the urban environment. These programs advocated strengthening the capacity of local authorities and community-based organizations; encouraging participatory processes, transparency, and accountability in government administration; and increasing the involvement of the private sector and civil society in all spheres of local activity.

Rethinking solutions to global challenges

Future urban transport studio

We are not alone in calling for essential changes in the academy in order to train future generations of researchers and practitioners to effectively meet the challenges of the current wave of global urbanisation and join with impoverished communities in addressing their self-identified health, social and environmental needs (Dalton, 2001; Durning, 2004; Mitrany and Stokols, 2005; Sclar et al, 2005b; Suarez-Balcazar et al, 2005). Towards this end, one mechanism we have recently instituted at Columbia University is the international and interdisciplinary Urban Planning Program studio (see www.arch.columbia.edu/UP/studios/studios.htm#studios). These real-world studios are taught by resident and invited faculty and are intended to familiarise students with interdisciplinary teamwork, data collection and analysis, and planning under time pressure.

In spring 2006, a future urban transport Urban Planning Program studio was held in Nairobi, Kenya, and conducted by Elliott D. Sclar in collaboration with faculty and students at the Center for Sustainable Urban Development, the

Mailman School of Public Health and the University of Nairobi. It focused on the Ruiru municipality within the larger Nairobi metropolitan area, which is located adjacent to and northeast of the Nairobi city limits.

In our view, every city is a solution to a transportation problem. Moreover, how we lay out our cities determines who has worse access and who has better access to employment, education, healthcare and other amenities. Thus, transport is more than an infrastructure – it is social policy.

Slum dwellers generally walk, bicycle or use collective modes of transit (Garau et al, 2005). According to Task Force 8 members (Garau et al, 2005, p 57):

> Sometimes even bicycles are out of reach. Lack of capital to buy shelter equipped with running water, sewerage, and pavement, in a location near jobs and public services, translates into a perpetual mobility burden. Safe, convenient, and reliable mobility is necessary for routine activities of daily living, such as traveling to work or shopping areas, as well as during crises....

Ecological framework

Figure 4.1 presents an ecological framework for thinking about future urban transport in Nairobi, Kenya that accounts for multiple levels of influence over time and space. It was adapted from previous conceptual models we developed for understanding determinants of population health and well-being at various scales or levels of influence (Northridge et al, 2003; Schulz and Northridge, 2004; Spielman et al, 2006). Here it has been modified to specifically examine relationships among gender and social inequalities at the societal level, the built environment and social context at the community level, stressors and buffers at the interpersonal level and disparities in health and well-being at the individual and population levels.

Fundamental (society) level

Starting with the column on the left side of the page, Figure 4.1 posits that the natural environment (including air quality, climate, and water supply), macro-social factors (including historical conditions; ideologies such as sexism, social justice and democracy; legal codes; economic orders; and human rights doctrines) and inequalities (including those related to the distribution of material wealth, employment and educational opportunities, and political influence) are *fundamental factors*. These broad societal factors underlie and influence both individual and population health and well-being via multiple pathways through differential access to power, information and resources (Link and Phelan, 1995), and are especially resistant to change, with notable exceptions, such as global climate change and human rights declarations.

Figure 4.1: Ecological model of future urban transport in Nairobi, Kenya

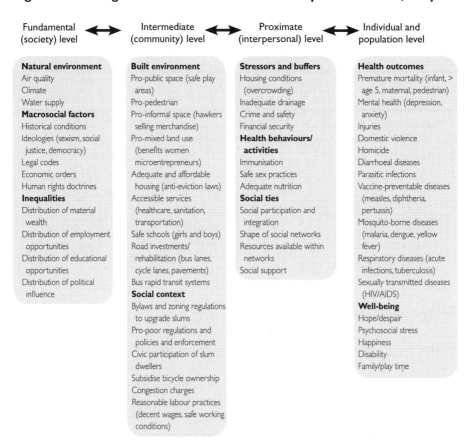

Note: This ecological framework for thinking about future urban transport in Nairobi, Kenya is adapted from a conceptual model that was developed for an article by Schulz and Northridge (2004). It has been modified to specifically examine relationships among gender and social inequalities at the societal level, the built environment and social context at the community level, stressors and buffers at the interpersonal level, and disparities in health and well-being at the individual and population levels.

Intermediate (community) level

Fundamental factors in turn influence *intermediate factors*, comprised in our model of both the built environment and social context. As a first pass, we have included under *built environment*:

- features that are pro-public space, such as safe play areas;
- features that are pro-pedestrian, such as traffic-calming engineering devices;
- features that are pro-informal space, so that, for example, hawkers can sell merchandise on streets;
- features that are pro-mixed land use, which, for example, benefits women microentrepreneurs;

- adequate and affordable housing, to include anti-eviction laws;
- accessible services, particularly healthcare, sanitation and transportation;
- safe schools to educate both girls and boys;
- road investments and rehabilitation measures, including bus lanes, bicycle lanes and pavements; and
- bus rapid transit systems.

Similarly, we have tentatively included under *social context* the following items:

- bylaws and zoning regulations to upgrade slums;
- pro-poor regulations and policies, along with the capacity and political will to enforce them;
- civic participation of slum dwellers, in order to end the green–brown divide between those with access to and those who are excluded from political and economic processes;
- subsidised bicycle ownership or formation of buyers' cooperatives of independent bicycle dealers to bring down the cost and improve the quality of bicycles;
- congestion charges, which benefit lower-income commuters; and
- reasonable labour practices, notably decent wages and safe working conditions for bus operators (Garau et al, 2005).

It is on such *intermediate factors* that we place particular emphasis, as intervening at the community level through non-health sector policies and programmes may have the greatest potential benefit for sustained improvements in population health and well-being, since they tend to be more structural rather than programme dependent. Indeed, urban planners work at the interface between the built environment and social context, applying the knowledge of social science and urban design to generate the physical configurations of cities.

Proximate (interpersonal) level

The more *proximate factors* influencing health and well-being are depicted in Figure 4.1 as stressors and buffers (including housing conditions such as overcrowding, inadequate drainage, crime and safety, and financial security), health behaviours and activities (including immunisation, safe sex practices and adequate nutrition) and social ties (including social participation and integration, the shape of social networks, the resources available within these networks and social support). Over the past several decades, public health research and practice has focused most often on influencing health behaviours and activities. If there is an absence of policy change at the intermediate level, however, such programmes are vulnerable and unlikely to be sustained.

Individual- and population-level health and well-being

Finally, the last column in the conceptual model represents *individual- and population-level health and well-being*, and lists a range of health outcomes that beset slum dwellers in Nairobi, Kenya (Zulu et al, 2002; Taffa, 2003; Amuyunzu-Nyamongo and Taffa, 2004; Borus, 2004; Gulis et al, 2004; Chakaya et al, 2005; Thuita et al, 2005). These health and well-being outcomes may include but are not limited to:

- premature mortality, including key indicators such as infant mortality, under age five childhood mortality, maternal mortality, and pedestrian mortality;
- mental health conditions, such as depression and anxiety;
- injuries across the lifecourse from falls, traffic and burns;
- domestic violence;
- homicide and suicide;
- diarrhoeal diseases, especially among youths;
- parasitic infections (worms);
- vaccine-preventable diseases, especially measles, diphtheria and pertussis;
- mosquito-borne diseases, notably malaria, dengue and yellow fever;
- respiratory diseases, both acute infections and chronic infections such as tuberculosis; and
- sexually transmitted diseases, including HIV/AIDS.

We also believe that it is essential to pay heed to relevant measures of well-being. Both well-being and its measures have heretofore been overly neglected in most public health frameworks. Hence, we have tentatively included hope and despair, psychosocial stress, happiness, disability and family and play time, as these clearly affect civic life across time and place. Still to be developed are culturally apt instruments to validly and reliably assess and monitor measures of well-being in Nairobi, Kenya.

Reinventing healthy and sustainable communities: an emphasis on process

Throughout this chapter, there has been an undercurrent of emphasis on process. All four of the transferable best principles outlined here were evident in the case study from Nairobi, Kenya. *Interdisciplinary engagement* helped us to conceive of the conceptual model on future urban transport presented in Figure 4.1. What is needed to develop it further at the local level is the active participation of Ruiru residents, government agencies and private investors. With explicit attention to *gender equality* and thoughtful consideration of the pathways that lead to improved population health and well-being for the urban poor, synergies may well result that lead to *sustainable development* and *democratic institution building*. Scaled up, these transferable best principles applied across sites may effectively address the urban challenge of slums and cities and thereby help in achieving the MDGs.

In order to reinvent healthy and sustainable communities, processes must be put in place to ensure that existing informal and slum settlements are upgraded and that adequate and affordable housing is built. Growing evidence suggests that community-led interventions designed and executed with the active participation of impoverished groups and their organisations can reduce costs and produce sustainable outcomes (Garau et al, 2005). We join Task Force 8 members in exhorting governments and international agencies not to lead, but rather to take their cues from the urban poor and place them as the drivers of their own futures.

In their book entitled *Prescription for a healthy nation: A new approach to improving our lives by fixing our everyday world*, Tom Farley and Deborah Cohen (2005) make the case that our built environments and social structures are responsible for 'humans behaving badly', that is, behaviours that lead to poor health. If we are to restructure our world and create 'healthscapes' rather than slums, we need to enlist visionary urban planners. This is why we approach our joint public health and urban planning initiatives from the ground up and focus on specific projects and experiences that make a difference in the health and welfare of the populations we serve. And this is why we encourage our students to keep asking the big questions (Northridge, forthcoming).

Acknowledgements

The authors thank Julie Touber and Nicole Volakva for their contributions to the future urban transport case study and suggestions for strengthening the attendant conceptual model, and Traci Bethea for her critical reading of the final draft of the chapter and attention to the references.

References

Amuyunzu-Nyamongo, M. and Taffa, N. (2004) 'The triad of poverty, environment and child health in Nairobi informal settlements', *Journal of Health and Population in Developing Countries*, January, www.povertyenvironment.net/?q=the_triad_of_poverty_environment_and_child_health_in_nairobi_informal_settlements (accessed 26 December 2008).

Arnstein, S.R. (1969) 'A ladder of citizen participation', *American Institute of Planners Journal* 35(4): 216-24.

Borus, P.K. (2004) 'Missed opportunities and inappropriately given vaccines reduce immunization coverage in facilities that serve slum areas of Nairobi', *East African Medical Journal* 81(3): 124-9.

Brownson, R.C., Chang, J.J., Eyler, A.A., Ainsworth, B.A., Kirtland, K.A., Saelens, B.E., and Sallis, J.F. (2004) 'Measuring the environment for friendliness toward physical activity: a comparison of the reliability of 3 questionnaires', *American Journal of Public Health* 94(3): 473-83.

Burrus, B., Northridge, M.E., Hund, L., Green, M., Braithwaite, K., Sabol, B., Healton, C. and Treadwell, H.M. for the Legacy/Community Voices Initiative (2006) 'Perspectives from the front lines of tobacco control', *Journal of Health Care for the Poor and Underserved* 17: 124–37.

Chakaya, J.M., Meme, H., Kwamanga, D., Githui, W.A., Onyango-Ouma, W.O., Gicheha, C., Karimi, F., Mansoer, J. and Kutwa, A. (2005) 'Planning for PPM-DOTS implementation in urban slums in Kenya: knowledge, attitude and practices of private health care providers in Kibera Slum, Nairobi', *The International Journal of Tuberculosis and Lung Disease* 9(4): 403–8.

Corburn, J. (2004) 'Confronting the challenges in reconnecting urban planning and public health', *American Journal of Public Health* 94(4): 541–6.

Dalton, L.C. (2001) 'Weaving the fabric of planning as education', *Journal of Planning Education and Research* 20(4): 423–36.

Dannenberg, A.L., Jackson, R.J., Frumkin, H., Schieber, R.A., Pratt, M., Kochtitzky, C. and Tilson, H.H.(2003) 'The impact of community design and land-use choices on public health: a scientific research agenda', *American Journal of Public Health* 93: 1500–8.

Darity, W. (2003) 'Will the poor always be with us?', *Review of Social Economy* LXI(4): 471–7.

Durning, B. (2004) 'Planning academics and planning practitioners: two tribes or a community of practice?' *Planning Practice and Research* 19(4): 435–46.

Fainstein, S.S. and Servon, L.J. (2005) (eds) *Gender and planning: A reader*, Piscataway, NJ: Rutgers University Press.

Farley, T. and Cohen, D.A. (2005) *Prescription for a healthy nation: A new approach to improving our lives by fixing our everyday world*, Boston, MA: Beacon Press.

Freudenberg, N. (2000) 'Health promotion in the city: a review of current practice and future prospects in the United States', *Annual Review of Public Health* 21: 473–503.

Frumkin, H. (2003) 'Healthy places: exploring the evidence', *American Journal of Public Health* 93: 1451–6.

Galea, S. and Vlahov, D. (2005) 'Urban health: evidence, challenges, and directions', *Annual Review of Public Health* 26: 341–65.

Garau, P., Sclar, E.D., and Carolini, G.Y., lead authors for the Task Force on Improving the Lives of Slum Dwellers (2005) *A home in the city: Achieving the millennium development goals*, London: Earthscan.

Gulis, G., Mulumba, J.A., Juma, O. and Kakosova, B. (2004) 'Health status of people of slums in Nairobi, Kenya', *Environmental Research* 96(2): 219–27.

Hoehner, C.M., Brennan, L.K., Brownson, R.C., Handy, S.L. and Killingsworth, R. (2003) 'Opportunities for integrating public health and urban planning approaches to promote active community environments', *American Journal of Health Promotion* 18(1):14–20.

Kaplan, S. and Kaplan, R. (2003) 'Health, Supportive environments and the reasonable person model', *American Journal of Public Health* 93(9): 1484–9.

Krieger, N. (2001) 'A glossary for social epidemiology', *International Journal of Epidemiology* 55: 693–700.

Link, B. G. and Phelan, J. 1995. 'Social conditions as fundamental causes of disease', *Journal of Health and Social Behavior*, Special issue: 80–94.

Macintyre, S., Ellaway, A., and Cummins, S. (2002) 'Place effects on health: how can we conceptualize, operationalize and measure them?' *Social Science and Medicine* 55: 125–39.

Mitrany, M. and Stokols, D. (2005) 'Gauging the transdisciplinary qualities and outcomes of doctoral training programs', *Journal of Planning Education and Research* 24(4): 437–49.

Nieves, A.D. (2002) '"With them the pen must be mightier than the sword": writing, engendering, and racializing planning history', *Journal of Planning History* 1(3): 215–19.

Northridge, M.E. (forthcoming) Book review of *Planet of slums* by Mike Davis, *Global Public Health*.

Northridge, M.E. and Sclar, E.D. (2002) 'Housing and health', *American Journal of Public Health* 92(5): 72.

Northridge, M.E. and Sclar, E. (2003) 'A joint urban planning and public health framework: contributions to health impact assessment', *American Journal of Public Health* 93(1): 118–21.

Northridge, M.E., Sclar, E.D. and Biswas, P. (2003) 'Sorting out the connections between the built environment and health: a conceptual framework for navigating pathways and planning healthy cities', *Journal of Urban Health* 80(4): 556–68.

Northridge, M.E., Shoemaker, K., Jean-Louis, B., Ortiz, B., Swaner, R., Vaughan, R.D., Cushman, L.F., Hutchinson, V.E., and Nicholas, S. (2005) 'What matters to communities? Using community-based participatory research to ask and answer questions regarding the environment and health. Essays on the future of environmental health research: a tribute to Dr. Kenneth Olden', *Environmental Health Perspective* 113(Suppl 1): 34–41.

Sallis, J.F., Frank, L.D., Saelens, B.E. and Kraft, M.K. (2004) 'Active transportation and physical activity: opportunities for collaboration on transportation and public health research', *Transportation Research Part A* 38: 249–68.

Schulz, A. and Northridge, M.E. (2004) 'Social determinants of health: implications for environmental health promotion', *Health, Education, and Behavior* 31(4): 455–71.

Sclar, E.D. and Northridge, M.E. (2001) 'Property, politics, and public health', *American Journal of Public Health* 91(7): 1013–15.

Sclar, E.D. and Northridge, M.E. (2003) 'Slums, slum dwellers, and health', *American Journal of Public Health* 93: 1381.

Sclar, E.D. and Touber, J. (2006) 'Future urban transport and achieving the millenium development goals: some lessons from Nairobi', Goteborg, Sweden: Third Future Urban Transport Conference, April.

Sclar, E.D., Garau, P. and Carolina, C. (2005a) 'The 21st century health challenge of slums and cities', *The Lancet* 365(9462): 901–3.

Sclar, E.D., Northridge, M.E., and Karpel, E.M. (2005b) 'Promoting interdisciplinary curricula and training in transportation, land use, physical activity, and health', Paper prepared for the Transportation Research Board and the Institute of Medicine Committee on Physical Activity, Health, Transportation, and Land Use, http://trb.org/downloads/sr282papers/sr282SclarNorthridgeKarpel.pdf (accessed 26 December 2008)

Spence, J.C. and Leeb, R.E. (2003) 'Toward a comprehensive model of physical activity', *Psychology of Sport and Exercise* 4: 7-24.

Spielman, S.E., Golembeski, C.A., Northridge, M.E., Vaughan, R.D., Swaner, R., Jean-Louis, B., Shoemaker, K., Klihr-Beall, S., Polley, E., Cushman, L.F., Ortiz, B., Hutchinson, V.E., Nicholas, S.W., Marx, T., Hayes, R., Goodman, A. and Sclar, E.D. (2006) 'Interdisciplinary planning for healthier communities: findings from the Harlem Children's Zone asthma initiative', *Journal of the American Planning Association*. 72(1): 100-8.

Srinivasan, S., O'Fallon, L.R. and Dearry A. (2003) 'Creating healthy communities, healthy homes, healthy people: initiating a research agenda on the built environment and public health', *American Journal of Public Health* 93: 1446-50.

Stephens, C., Akerman, M., Avle, S., Borlina Maia, P., Campanario, P., Doe, B. and Tetteh, D. (1997) 'Urban equity and urban health: using existing data to understand inequalities in health and environment in Accra, Ghana and Sao Paulo, Brazil', *Environment and Urbanization* 9(1): 181-202.

Suarez-Balcazar, Y., Harper, G.W., and Lewis, R. (2005) 'An interactive and contextual model of community–university collaborations for research and action', *Health Education Behavior* 32(1): 84-101.

Taffa, N. (2003) 'A comparison of pregnancy and child health outcomes between teenage and adult mothers in the slums of Nairobi, Kenya', *The International Journal of Adolescent Medical Health* 15(4): 321-9.

Thuita, F.M., Mwadime, R.K. and Wang'ombe, J.K. (2005) 'Child nutritional status and maternal factors in an urban slum in Nairobi, Kenya', *East African Medical Journal* 82(4): 209-15.

TRB (Transportation Research Board) and Institute of Medicine of the National Academies (eds) (2005) *Does the built environment influence physical activity? Examining the evidence*, Special Report 282, Washington, DC: TRB.

UN Population Division (1999) *World Urbanization Prospectus*, New York, NY: UN Population Division.

Yang, P.Q. (2000) *Ethnic studies: Issues and approaches*, New York, NY: State University of New York Press.

Zulu, E.M., Dodoo, F.N. and Chika-Ezee, A. (2002) 'Sexual risk-taking in the slums of Nairobi, Kenya, 1993–8', *Population Studies* 56(3): 311-23.

Pathway 2
Group advantage and disadvantage

How and why do interventions that increase health overall widen inequalities within populations?

Martin White, Jean Adams and Peter Heywood

Introduction

Health inequalities between groups within populations defined by place of residence, race, ethnicity or culture, occupation, gender, religion, age, education, income or other measure of socioeconomic position (SEP) are widely observed (Marmot et al, 1978; Townsend and Davidson, 1982; Charlton and White, 1995) and, in many contexts, growing (Adams et al, 2006). Reducing health inequalities has become an important objective of governments worldwide (US Department of Health and Human Services, 2000; Department of Health, 2004). However, evidence for strategies to reduce health inequalities is limited and systematic reviews have failed to offer substantive analyses or contribute to theory (Arblaster et al, 1996; Gunning-Schepers and Gepkens, 1996). Health inequities are inequalities or differences in health between populations or groups within populations that are considered unfair and avoidable (Kawachi et al, 2002; Macinko and Starfield, 2002). The term 'inequality' is used throughout this chapter, although it is impossible to make the necessary value judgements to designate observed differences as 'unfair and avoidable' in the space available, nor is it central to the arguments presented here.

Contemporary health strategies at international, national and local levels share the twin aims of improving overall health and reducing inequalities in health between groups within the population. Although common sense may suggest that these aims should be achievable in tandem, an intervention that improves the health of a population overall may also increase inequalities in health (Macintyre, 2000; Victora et al, 2000; Mechanic, 2002; Tugwell et al, 2006).

Variations in the provision of, and response to, many interventions according to SEP have been noted and, to date, have generally been described in terms of the 'inverse care law' (ICL) (Tudor Hart, 1971). However, the ICL narrowly describes variations in provision of medical care according to need, not variations in effectiveness of a range of interventions according to SEP. In this chapter, we review past attempts to theorise this problem and present evidence suggesting that inequalities can be introduced at all stages of the planning and delivery of interventions that affect health. When such inequalities are patterned according to socioeconomic variables, they may be due to reliance of interventions on voluntary behaviour change and other limitations of intervention design. Conversely, strategies that use regulation (resulting in compulsory behaviour change) or incentives (leading to discrete resource gains) may have beneficial effects on socioeconomic equity. The widespread nature and implications of such inequalities generated by interventions makes them of importance to policy makers, practitioners and researchers of all disciplines. Systematic approaches are required to research and tackle this apparently universal phenomenon.

Background: 'inverse' laws and the equity–effectiveness trade-off

The inverse care law

The ICL states that 'the availability of good medical care tends to vary inversely with the need for it in the population served' (Tudor Hart, 1971, p 405). As health and the need for healthcare are closely associated with SEP, the ICL has been interpreted to suggest that the most socioeconomically deprived communities will have the least access to good-quality medical care. Although the ICL originally focused on the provision of primary healthcare, the term has now been applied to a variety of aspects of healthcare including service utilisation (Webb, 1998), length of consultation (Stirling et al, 2001), willingness of general practitioners to prescribe antidepressants (Chew-Graham et al, 2002), satisfaction with antenatal care (Brown and Lumley, 1997) and use of health-promotion services (Wright, 1997). In general, these non-specific applications of the ICL focus on socioeconomic deprivation, rather than absolute need for services, and rarely identify that they are using socioeconomic deprivation as a marker of need for services. Because of this widespread, loose interpretation of the ICL, the meaning of the term has become increasingly confused and non-specific, although its appeal as a rhetorical device has not diminished (Watt, 2002). This is perhaps surprising, since it was conceived in a 'rambling polemic', with no empirical basis, no testable explanatory framework, and no suggestions for ways to intervene (Watt, 2002).

The inverse prevention law and inverse equity hypothesis

Recently, there have been a number of formal attempts to develop the idea underlying the ICL for a wider range of health interventions – in particular, preventive and population-level strategies. The concept of the 'inverse prevention law' was no more than a throwaway line in the influential UK government's Acheson Report on health inequalities, published in 1999 (Acheson, 2000). It alluded to the idea that there seems likely to be a concept analogous to the ICL for prevention, whereby those most likely to benefit from preventive measures (that is, those most at risk and, often, those living in the most deprived circumstances) tend to be least likely to receive them. While many would endorse this hypothesis, no evidence was produced to substantiate this claim in the report.

Victora et al (2000) provided an empirical basis for their proposed 'inverse equity hypothesis' (IEH), drawing on studies of child health in Brazil. The IEH, described as 'a corollary of the ICL', identifies the process by which new public health interventions lead to an initial widening of socioeconomic inequalities, due to preferential uptake by the most advantaged, before inequality narrows and overall health improves, due to subsequent uptake by the less advantaged groups in the population. This 'trickle-down' effect was subsequently attributed to the theory of diffusion of innovations (Rodgers, 2003; Schellenberg et al, 2003). Building on the initial concept in a subsequent paper, Victora et al (2003) expand their explanation to suggest that there are multiple ways in which the poorest may be disadvantaged. They use this to explain that the poorest suffer from compound disadvantages such as reduced host resistance through poor nutrition, greater exposure to risks and reduced access to health interventions through lower educational attainment and greater levels of illiteracy, as well as poorer-quality services because few professionals wish to work in the poorest areas (Schellenberg et al, 2003). The IEH remains a general theory developed for low-income countries with no specification of causal pathways, and thus does not identify specific ways to intervene (apart from 'universal coverage' with health resources), nor provide supportive evidence for interventions to reduce 'inverse equity'.

The equity–effectiveness loop

In 1985 Tugwell and colleagues suggested that effectiveness of (clinical) interventions should be looked at iteratively because many stages in the intervention process may contribute to overall or 'community' effectiveness (Tugwell et al, 1985). More recently, Tugwell and colleagues suggested that the potential existed for inequality to be introduced at different stages in clinical systems (Tugwell et al, 2006). In other words, the efficacy of an intervention in different socioeconomic groups may be modified by equity of access to the intervention, diagnostic accuracy, provider compliance and consumer adherence, all contributing to differential overall effectiveness by SEP. This framework suggests a systematic method for exploring the relationship between effectiveness and equity, although does not distinguish clearly between provision of an intervention and responses to it, and thus ignores some important points at which inequalities could be introduced. A 'staircase' effect is proposed, whereby factors that modify efficacy do so in a multiplicative way, leading to an estimate of community effectiveness that is the product of efficacy and each successive modifier. To take an example, an intervention may be efficacious in 50% of those to whom it is delivered appropriately, but the condition for which it is efficacious is only diagnosed in 80% of those with the condition, only 60% of those diagnosed gain access to the intervention, only 90%

of providers deliver the intervention as intended and only 70% of consumers adhere to the intervention as intended. Its overall community effectiveness will thus be the product of the efficacy, multiplied by each of these modifiers (that is, $0.5 \times 0.8 \times 0.6 \times 0.9 \times 0.7 = 0.15$). In other words, the intervention would have an overall community effectiveness in 15% of the target population. Furthermore, if the magnitude of any of these five modifiers of the efficacy of the intervention varied by SEP, then a socioeconomic gradient of effectiveness would be observed. Tugwell et al present no direct evidence to support a multiplicative effect and it is possible that modifying factors affect efficacy in different (mathematical) ways.

Tugwell et al's (2006) paper suggests some intervention examples (for example social marketing to promote chemical impregnated bed nets for malaria prevention), but does not identify key characteristics of interventions that may widen or narrow inequalities, suggesting that this will be the role of the newly formed Cochrane Collaboration Equity Field.

Intervention-generated inequalities and outcome gradients

The theories presented above, when considered together, suggest that *all* processes in the planning and delivery of an intervention have the potential to widen inequalities between groups within the target population, distinguished by a range of factors, such as gender, age, ethnicity or SEP. (We have used the term 'intervention-generated inequalities' throughout to describe unequal outcomes of any stage of an intervention process. The term 'iatrogenic' could be used in cases where these inequalities are introduced by a doctor, but is too specific a term to use in all cases.) Inequalities between groups, while individually small, may act additively or multiplicatively (or in other mathematical relationships), leading to significant and measurable inequalities in final outcomes. Such potential inequalities seem likely to occur in all public sectors and systems (for example education – Losen and Orfield, 2002 – and criminal justice – Free, 2004), although we only present evidence for health systems here. Similarly, although evidence exists for such effects in relation to ethnicity or race (van Ryn and Fu, 2003) and gender (Raine et al, 2003) (and we assume place, religion and age), we focus here on evidence for intervention-generated inequalities by SEP, measured by factors such as educational attainment, occupational class and income.

Figure 5.1 identifies key stages in the intervention process at which inequalities can be introduced and illustrates these with examples relating to cardiovascular disease. The provision of interventions to improve health includes the processes involved in assessing needs for services and specific interventions. Intervention-generated inequalities could occur, for example, when a community survey is used to assess the need for a specific intervention. Socioeconomic variations in response rates (Turrell et al, 2002) may lead to underestimation of need in the most socially disadvantaged groups. Similarly, poorer groups and those from minority ethnic groups are often less well represented in trials and other evaluative

Figure 5.1: Points during the planning and delivery of interventions to prevent and treat cardiovascular disease where socioeconomic outcome inequalities might occur, and examples of reported inequalities

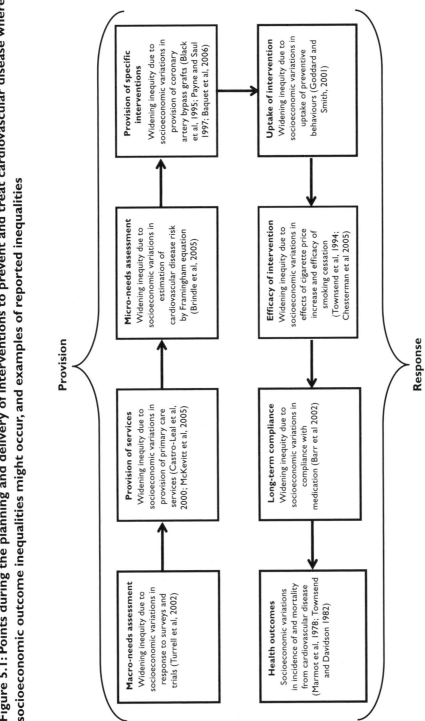

studies, leading to bias in assessment of outcome effects across the socioeconomic spectrum (Baquet et al, 2006).

Research that does not control for the potential confounding effects of SEP can lead to false conclusions (von Elm and Egger, 2004). It has also been reported that the Framingham equation (a cardiovascular risk score) underestimates cardiovascular mortality risk more in manual, compared to non-manual, groups (Brindle et al, 2005) and the Rose Angina Questionnaire elicits different responses from people of different ethnic origin in the UK (Fischbacher et al, 2001). Likewise, there is evidence that both services in general and specific interventions are delivered unequally, with the benefit in favour of more affluent groups (Scott et al, 1996; Castro-Leal et al, 2000; Goddard and Smith, 2001; Chew-Graham et al, 2002; Saxena et al, 2002; Hetemaa et al, 2003; McKevitt et al, 2005; Milner et al, 2004; Morris et al, 2005; Morris and Landes, 2006). Importantly, this extends to the offer of preventive interventions, in particular in primary healthcare (Kaner et al, 2001; Houston et al, 2005; Qi et al, 2006).

Individuals may also respond to health interventions in a manner that increases social inequalities in health. For example, there are well-documented socioeconomic variations in uptake of a number of public health interventions, including physician visits (Virtanen et al, 2006), cancer screening (Qi et al, 2006), screening for Down's syndrome (Dormandy et al, 2005), immunisations (Reading et al, 1994), correct use of folic acid pre-conception to prevent neural tube defects (Relton et al, 2005) and breast feeding (Kirk, 1980). Use of safety equipment, such as seatbelts (Colgan et al, 2003) and bicycle helmets (Farley et al, 1996), is also often socioeconomically patterned as is compliance with therapeutic interventions (Barr et al, 2002).

Efficacy of interventions can also be socially patterned. Econometric models predict that traditional interventions to reduce cigarette smoking, such as health education and smoking restrictions, are likely to have the greatest effect among more affluent smokers (Townsend et al, 1994). Evidence also suggests that smoking cessation interventions are less effective among more socially deprived groups (Chesterman et al, 2005). In two studies charting the effects of the 'Back To Sleep' campaign to prevent sudden infant deaths in the 1990s, significantly lower responses to the educational intervention were demonstrated among poorer and minority ethnic families in the UK (Blair et al, 2006) and the US (Pickett et al, 2005). In a study evaluating the effects of bicycle helmet legislation in Canada, despite a sizeable initial effect on all social groups, narrowing the pre-existing socioeconomic inequality, six years after the legislation was introduced the effect was sustained in the more affluent but not the more deprived social groups, resulting in wider inequality than before the intervention (Macpherson et al, 2006). This result suggests that the overall effectiveness and equity of an intervention may vary with time following the intervention.

While the majority of stages of the provision of, and responses to, a health intervention (as shown in Figure 5.1) might be expected to lead to increased social inequalities in health, it is also possible that unequal outcomes of steps in any intervention process can favour the deprived rather than the affluent and so reduce inequality, as illustrated in Figure 5.2. Examples include the effect of water fluoridation on child dental health (Jones and Worthington, 1999), legislation on bicycle helmet use (Parkin et al, 2003) and price increases on cigarette smoking (Townsend et al, 1994). There is also some evidence that financial incentives to general practitioners lead to decreased socioeconomic inequalities in cervical screening and childhood immunisations (Baker and Middleton, 2003). Financial incentives targeting individuals may also reduce pre-existing socioeconomic inequalities (Harland et al, 1999).

Thus, within any single planning and delivery pathway, socioeconomic gradients may oppose one another at different stages, and theoretically even cancel each other out. However, in most cases it is more likely that they are typically cumulative, such that small socioeconomic gradients in the same direction at each step combine (for example, additively or multiplicatively, or in another mathematical relationship) to produce the substantial socioeconomic gradients in morbidity and mortality that have been widely measured (Tugwell et al's so-called 'staircase' effect; Tugwell et al, 2006). The nature and magnitude of such cumulative effects are likely to vary from case to case and require empirical evaluation. In proposing this idea we have, for simplicity, assumed that socioeconomic gradients are linear. While this is often the case, it is not always so and more complex relationships may also exist.

Interventions may also have unexpected side effects and these might have a greater impact on some population groups than others. For example, the introduction of a school-based bicycle safety education programme paradoxically led to more bicycling-related injuries, especially among the poorest children. This may have been due to inadvertent encouragement of risk-taking (Carlin et al, 1998). Methods are needed to explore such inequitable side effects of interventions, as well as the main (intended) effects.

Characteristics of interventions that increase or decrease socioeconomic inequalities

A common attribute of interventions that lead to increased socioeconomic inequalities in health appears to be a reliance on voluntary behaviour change (Mechanic, 2002). Thus, for example, although governed by law, ultimately the decision to wear a seatbelt rests with the individual, leading to a social patterning in seatbelt wearing (Colgan et al, 2003). Likewise, although we might intend that a policy to screen all women aged over 50 for breast cancer should apply equally to all women, without some compulsion to attend, uptake of screening remains voluntary and can result in inequality (Adams et al, 2004). While such factors may be a key source of socioeconomic inequalities, it is important to recognise that health-related choices might not be entirely 'free' or independent in every situation. Nor should choice necessarily be removed from public health interventions (Nuffield Council on Bioethics, 2007) – but it should be recognised as a potentially important cause of widening inequalities.

Figure 5.2: Schematic representation of potential socioeconomic outcome inequality gradients resulting from an intervention that affects health

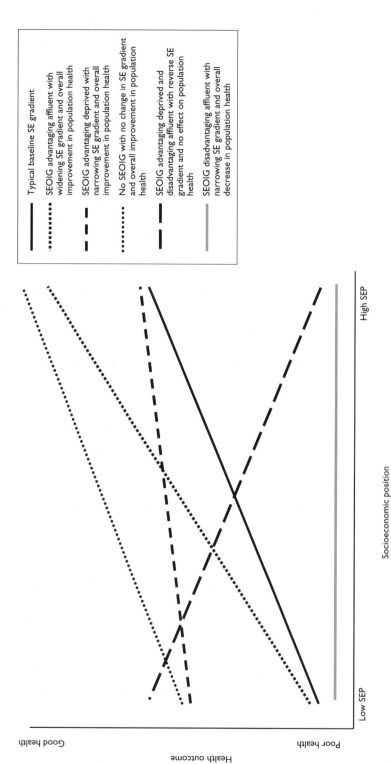

Note: SE=socioeconomic; SEOIG=socioeconomic outcome inequality gradient.

The example of water fluoridation illustrates what can happen when a public health intervention circumvents such a voluntary behaviour change (Mechanic, 2002). An obvious attribute of water fluoridation in a geographical area served by a single supply is that it is universally delivered and taken up, except perhaps by a very small number of people who choose to drink only bottled water or have their own well. However, although largely effective, water fluoridation does not entirely eradicate socioeconomic inequalities in dental health (Jones and Worthington, 1999) because fluoride is not the only determinant of dental health – sugar consumption and tooth brushing, both voluntary behaviours, also play a role and are socioeconomically patterned (Maliderou et al, 2006).

Other methods of delivering public health interventions that may circumvent reliance on voluntary behaviour change include financial incentives (Baker and Middleton, 2003) or disincentives (Townsend et al, 1994), making services more accessible to deprived groups (Baker and Middleton, 2003), or targeting interventions specifically at lower social groups (Krieger et al, 1999). This suggests that many structural factors can affect service use and that these may facilitate or curtail 'choice' in ways that may not be obvious or measurable. Evidence to support this comes from a number of studies where financial and material barriers to intervention effectiveness in poorer groups have been identified, including sudden infant death syndrome (continued bed sharing) (Blair et al, 2006), ability to afford bicycle helmets (Kendrick and Royal, 2003) and ability to afford up-front payments for elective surgery (Kaufman et al, 2006).

There are two important implications of these findings. The first is that to reduce inequalities as well as improve health, a single intervention modality (such as a policy that is not supported by education) may not be enough. Conversely, interventions that combine a range of methods, such as a policy measure, educational interventions, a technology and resource incentives, as seen for example in UK immunisation programmes (Department of Health, 2005), may help to reduce or avoid intervention-generated inequalities. Second, interventions that are delivered in the same way to all recipients may result in differential outcomes. Resultant inequalities may be, for example, because the less affluent or educated are less able to access the intervention, understand it or engage with it. The problem with 'one-size-fits-all' interventions has been recognised (Ashworth, 1997; Bull et al, 1999; Adams and White, 2007) and is likely to be another characteristic of interventions that may widen inequality. The corollary of this is that interventions that are tailored for the needs of individuals or subgroups within a target population may be more likely to result in outcomes that are more equitable, and there is evidence to support this supposition (Marcus et al, 1998; Panter-Brick et al, 2006). The specific effects of each intervention component need to be evaluated quantitatively to confirm this hypothesis.

Implications for policy, practice and research

The potential for any or all stages in the planning and delivery of interventions that affect health to generate or widen socioeconomic inequalities means that policy makers, practitioners and researchers should be aware of them and the implications they may have. Those developing policy and planning services should be aware of the socioeconomic biases in who responds to consultative exercises and who lobbies for change, and the potential for inequitable effects of interventions. The techniques of prospective health equity impact assessment (Douglas and Scott-Samuel, 2001) are evolving and could be routinely used to assess the potential for any element or stage of an intervention to result in widening inequality. Those delivering services should be aware of socioeconomic variations in uptake and outcome of therapeutic or preventive interventions. The techniques of health equity audit (Hamer et al, 2005), closely related to health equity impact assessment, could be routinely employed by professionals implementing and monitoring interventions in practice. Those trialling and implementing health interventions should be alert to the possibility that adherence and efficacy may vary according to SEP. To this end, we believe that investigating the effect of health interventions according to SEP should become a routine aspect of intervention evaluation, a proposal now endorsed by the Cochrane and Campbell collaborations (Tugwell et al, 2006).

Although we have focused here on socioeconomic inequalities, it is likely that similar cumulative differences in provision and response occur according to other variables such as gender, age and ethnic group (Raine et al, 2003; van Ryn and Fu, 2003). Researchers need to be aware of the meaning and relevance of different measures of SEP (such as education, income and social class) and, more generally, measures of 'difference' between population groups when researching the unequal outcomes of interventions. Furthermore, while most of the examples referred to here are from developed countries, it seems likely that the phenomenon of adverse outcome equity is universal (Castro-Leal et al, 2000; Victora et al, 2000; Schellenberg et al, 2003; Tugwell et al, 2006). Programmes of research are needed to assess the evidence for the theories discussed here, including systematic reviews of intervention equity, secondary analyses of existing trial and disease register data, and prospective studies of differential intervention effectiveness. Qualitative studies may also be needed to understand the processes leading to inequalities quantified in evaluative studies. The concept of socioeconomic, and other, intervention-generated inequalities therefore sets a wide-ranging agenda for health equity research.

One further consideration needs exploration. Tugwell et al (2006) refer to the trade-off between equity and effectiveness. However, in any health system we also trade off effectiveness against efficiency. For example, the National Institute for Health and Clinical Excellence (NICE) in the UK has a remit to identify not only the most effective, but also the most cost-effective interventions on which the National Health Service (NHS) should spend its scarce resources.

An inequitable outcome is sub-optimally effective, yet an intervention tailored to individual needs might be significantly more costly, as shown by smoking cessation services in the UK (Godfrey et al, 2005). Thus, there is also likely to be an implicit trade-off between equity and efficiency in much healthcare and public health decision making. The consequences of this are profound: we have to think about effectiveness, efficiency *and* equity routinely in intervention research; and we have to make explicit decisions about equity–effectiveness and equity–efficiency trade-offs in delivering public services. We also need to become more aware of the effects on equity of current policies within health systems, such as the strong current UK NHS focus on performance targets and efficiency (Bevan and Hood, 2006).

Conclusions

While the ICL identified an important aspect of the nature of healthcare, it has now been so widely and loosely interpreted as to become confusing. A number of theories have been proposed to extend the ideas that originated in the ICL, and others have contributed supportive evidence or ideas. In this chapter, we have attempted to synthesise this range of evidence and propose a framework for understanding, researching and tackling inequalities resulting from health interventions. A joint health equity group has recently been established by the Cochrane and Campbell collaborations (Tugwell et al, 2006). An important first task will be to define terminology, since none of the terms that have been proposed to replace ICL (Acheson, 1998; Victora et al, 2000; Tugwell et al, 2006) adequately describes the phenomenon, its consequences or approaches to understand or tackle it.

Practitioners, policy makers and researchers should be aware of the widespread potential for intervention-generated inequalities as they may bias a wide variety of results. Further research is required to clarify the causes of intervention inequalities, to determine their ability to account for social inequalities in health and, importantly, to identify cost-effective strategies to reduce or avoid them.

The widespread belief that the ICL cannot fully account for social inequalities in health, as exemplified by the Black Report's assessment that 'unequal usage of healthcare will never be more than a partial explanation' (Townsend and Davidson, 1982, p 76), may be the case. However, if socioeconomic inequalities at all stages of the planning and delivery of interventions that affect health are considered, it is likely that they will account statistically for a larger proportion of socioeconomic inequalities in health than the ICL alone. Taking this approach should ensure that addressing intervention-generated inequalities will become an important public health endeavour, as suggested by Derek Wanless (2004) in his report to the UK Treasury entitled *Securing good health for the whole population*.

References

Acheson, D. (1998) *Report of the independent inquiry into inequalities in health*, London: The Stationery Office.

Acheson, D. (2000) 'Health inequalities impact assessment', *Bulletin of the World Health Organization* 78: 75-6.

Adams, J. and White, M. (2007) 'Are the stages of change socio-economically patterned: a scoping review', *American Journal of Health Promotion* 21: 237-47.

Adams, J., Holland, L. and White, M. (2006) 'Changes in socioeconomic inequalities in census measures of health in England and Wales, 1991–2001', *Journal of Epidemiology & Community Health* 60: 218-20.

Adams, J., White, M. and Forman, D. (2004) 'Are there socio-economic gradients in stage and grade of breast cancer at diagnosis? A cross sectional analysis of UK cancer registry data', *British Medical Journal* 329: 142-3.

Arblaster, L., Lambert, M., Entwistle, V., Forster, M., Fullerton, D., Sheldon, T. and Watt, I. (1996) 'A systematic review of the effectiveness of health service interventions aimed at reducing inequalities in health', *Journal of Health Service Research & Policy* 1: 93-103.

Ashworth, P. (1997) 'Breakthrough or bandwagon? Are interventions tailored to Stage of Change more effective than non-staged interventions?', *Health Education Journal* 56: 166-74.

Baker, D. and Middleton, E. (2003) 'Cervical screening and health inequality in England in the 1990s', *Journal of Epidemiology & Community Health* 57: 417-23.

Baquet, C.R., Commiskey, P., Mullins, C.D. and Mishra, S.I. (2006) 'Recruitment and participation in clinical trials: socio-demographic, rural/urban, and health care access predictors', *Cancer Detection & Prevention* 30: 24-33.

Barr, R.G., Somers, S.C., Speizer, F.E. and Camargo, C.A. (2002) 'Patient factors and medication guidance adherence among older women with asthma', *Archives of Internal Medicine* 162: 1761-8.

Bevan, G. and Hood, C. (2006) 'Have targets improved performance in the English NHS?', *British Medical Journal* 332: 419-22.

Black, N., Langham, S. and Petticrew, M. (1995) 'Coronary revascularisation: why do rates vary geographically in the UK?', *Journal of Epidemiology & Community Health* 49: 408-12.

Blair, P.S., Sidebotham, P., Berry, P.J., Evans, M. and Fleming, P.J. (2006) 'Major epidemiological changes in sudden infant death syndrome: a 20-year population-based study in the UK', *The Lancet* 367: 314-19.

Brindle, P.M., McConnachie, A., Upton, M.N., Hart, C.L., Davey Smith, G. and Watt, G.C. (2005) 'The accuracy of the Framingham risk-score in different socioeconomic groups: a prospective study', *British Journal of General Practice* 55: 838-45.

Brown, S. and Lumley, J. (1997) 'Antenatal care: a case of the inverse care law?' *Australian Journal of Public Health* 17: 95-103.

Bull, F.C., Kreuter, M.W. and Scharff, D.P. (1999) 'Effects of tailored, personalized and general health messages on physical activity', *Patient Education & Counseling* 36: 181-92.

Carlin, J.B., Taylor, P. and Nolan, T. (1998) 'School based bicycle safety education and bicycle injuries in children: a case-control study', *Injury Prevention* 4: 22-7.

Castro-Leal, F., Dayton, J., Demery, L. and Mehra, K. (2000) 'Public spending on health care in Africa: do the poor benefit?', *Bulletin of the World Health Organization* 78: 66-74.

Charlton, B.G. and White, M. (1995) 'Living on the margin: a salutogenic model for socio-economic differentials in health', *Public Health* 109: 235-43.

Chesterman, J., Judge, K., Bauld, L. and Ferguson, J. (2005) 'How effective are the English smoking treatment services in reaching disadvantaged smokers?', *Addiction* 100: 36-45.

Chew-Graham, C.A., Mullin, S., May, C.R., Hedley, S. and Cole, H. (2002) 'Managing depression in primary care: another example of the inverse care law', *Family Practice* 19: 632-7.

Colgan, F., Gospel, A., Petrie, A., Adams, J., Heywood, P. and White, M. (2003) 'Is rear seatbelt use socio-economically distributed?', *Journal of Epidemiology & Community Health* 58: 929-30.

Department of Health (2004) *Choosing health: Making healthy choices easier*, London: HMSO.

Department of Health (2005) *Vaccination services: Reducing inequalities in uptake*, London: Department of Health .

Dormandy, E., Michie, S., Hooper, R. and Marteau, T.M. (2005) 'Low uptake of prenatal screening for Down's syndrome in minority ethnic groups and socially deprived groups: a reflection of women's attitudes or a failure to facilitate informed choices?', *International Journal of Epidemiology* 34: 346-52.

Douglas, M. and Scott-Samuel, A. (2001) 'Addressing health inequalities in health impact assessment', *Journal of Epidemiology & Community Health* 55: 450-1.

Farley, C., Haddad, S. and Brown, B. (1996) 'The effects of a 4-year program promoting bicycle helmet use among children in Quebec', *American Journal of Public Health* 86: 46-51.

Fischbacher, C.M., Bhopal, R.S., Unwin, N., White, M. and Alberti, K.G.M.M. (2001) 'The performance of the Rose angina questionnaire in South Asian and European populations: a comparative study in Newcastle, UK', *International Journal of Epidemiology* 30: 1009-16.

Free, M.D. (ed) (2004) *Racial issues in criminal justice: The case of African Americans*, Monsey, NY: Criminal Justice Press.

Goddard, M. and Smith, P. (2001) 'Equity of access to health care services: theory and evidence from the UK', *Social Science & Medicine* 53: 1149-62.

Godfrey, C., Parrott, S., Colemen, T. and Pound, E. (2005) 'The cost-effectiveness of the English smoking treatment services: evidence from practice', *Addiction* 100: 70-83.

Gunning-Schepers, L.J. and Gepkens, A. (1996) 'Reviews of interventions to reduce social inequalities in health: research and policy implications', *Health Education Research* 55: 226-38.

Hamer, L., Killoran, A., Macknight, A. and Falce, C. (2005) *Health equity audit: Learning from practice briefing*, London: NHS National Institute for Health and Clinical Excellence.

Harland, J.O.E., White, M., Drinkwater, C., Chinn, D., Farr, L. and Howel, D. (1999) 'The Newcastle Exercise Project: a randomised controlled trial of methods to promote physical activity in primary care', *British Medical Journal* 319: 828-32.

Hetemaa, T., Keskimaki, I., Manderbacka, A., Laeyland, A.H. and Koskinen, S. (2003) 'How did the recent increase in supply of coronary operations in Finland affect socio-economic and gender equity in their use?', *Journal of Epidemiology & Community Health* 57: 178-85.

Houston, T.K., Scarini, I.C., Person, S.D. and Greene, P.G. (2005) 'Patient smoking cessation advice by health care providers: the role of ethnicity, socio-economic status and health', *American Journal of Public Health* 95: 1056-61.

Jones, C. and Worthington, H. (1999) 'The relationship between water fluoridation and socio-economic deprivation on tooth decay in 5-year-old children', *British Dental Journal* 186: 397-400.

Kaner, E.F.S., Heather, N., Brodie, J., Lock, C.A. and McAvoy, B.R. (2001) 'Patient and practitioner characteristics predict brief alcohol intervention in primary care', *British Journal of General Practice* 51: 822-7.

Kaufman, W., Chavez, A.S., Skipper, B. and Kaufman, A. (2006) 'Effect of high up front charges on access to surgery for poor patients at a public hospital in Mexico', *International Journal for Equity in Health* 5: 6.

Kawachi, I., Subramanian, S.V. and Almeida-Filho, N. (2002) 'A glossary for health inequalities', *Journal of Epidemiology & Community Health* 56: 647-52.

Kendrick, D. and Royal, S. (2003) 'Inequalities in cycle helmet use: cross sectional survey in schools in deprived areas of Nottingham', *Archives of Diseases in Childhood* 88: 876-80.

Kirk, T. (1980) 'Appraisal of the effectiveness of nutrition education in the context of infant feeding', *Journal of Human Nutrition* 34: 429-38.

Krieger, M., Quesenberry, C., Peng, T., Horn-Ross, P., Stewart, S., Brown, S., Swallen, K., Guillermo, T., Suh, D., Alvarez-Martinez, L. and Ward, F. (1999) 'Social class, race/ethnicity, and incidence of breast, cervix, colon, lung, and prostate cancer among Asian, black, Hispanic, and white residents of the San Francisco Bay Area, 1988–92 (United States)', *Cancer Causes & Control* 10: 525-37.

Losen, D. and Orfield. G. (2002) *Racial inequity in special education*, Cambridge, MA: Harvard University Press.

Macinko, J.A. and Starfield, B. (2002) 'Annotated bibliography on equity in health', *International Journal for Equity in Health* 1: 1.

Macintyre, S. (2000) 'Prevention and the reduction of health inequalities', *British Medical Journal* 320: 1399-1400.

McKevitt, C., Coshall, C., Tilling, K. and Wolfe, C. (2005) 'Are there inequalities in the provision of stroke care? Analysis of an inner-city stroke register', *Stroke* 36: 315-20.

Macpherson, A.K., Macarthur, C., To, T.M., Chipman, M.L., Wright, J.G. and Parkin, P.C. (2006), 'Economic disparity in bicycle helmet use by children six years after the introduction of legislation', *Injury Prevention* 12: 231-5.

Maliderou, M., Reeves, S. and Noble, C. (2006) 'The effect of social demographic factors, snack consumption and vending machine use on oral health of children living in London', *British Dental Journal* 201: 441-4.

Marcus, B.H., Bock, B.C., Pinto, B.M., Forsyth, L.H., Roberts, M.B. and Traficante, R.M. (1998) 'Efficacy of an individualized, motivationally-tailored physical activity intervention', *Annals of Behavioral Medicine* 20: 174-80.

Marmot, M.G., Rose, G., Shipley, M. and Hamilton, P.J.S. (1978) 'Employment grade and coronary heart disease in British civil servants', *Journal of Epidemiology & Community Health* 32: 244-9.

Mechanic, D. (2002) 'Disadvantage, inequality, and social policy', *Health Affairs* 21: 48-59.

Milner, P.C., Payne, J.N., Stanfield, R.C., Lewis, P.A., Jennison, C. and Saul, C. (2004) 'Inequalities in accessing hip joint replacement for people in need', *European Journal of Public Health* 14: 58-62.

Morris, E. and Landes, D. (2006) 'The equity of access to orthodontic dental care for children in the North East of England', *Public Health* 120: 359-63.

Morris, S., Sutton, M. and Gravelle, H. (2005) 'Inequity and inequality in the use of health care in England: an empirical investigation', *Social Science & Medicine* 60: 1251-66.

Nuffield Council on Bioethics (2007) *Public health: Ethical issues*, Cambridge: Cambridge Publishers Ltd.

Panter-Brick, C., Clarke, S.E., Lomas, H., Pinder, M. and Lindsay, S.W. (2006)'Culturally compelling strategies for behaviour change: a social ecology model and case study in malaria prevention', *Social Science & Medicine* 62: 2810-25.

Parkin, P.C., Khambalia, A., Kmet, L. and Macarthur, C. (2003) 'Influence of socioeconomic status on the effectiveness of bicycle helmet legislation for children: a prospective observational study', *Pediatrics* 112: e192-e196.

Payne, N. and Saul, C. (1997) 'Variations in use of cardiology services in a health authority: comparison of coronary artery revascularisation rates with prevalence of angina and coronary mortality', *British Medical Journal* 314: 257.

Pickett, K.E., Luo, Y. and Lauderdale, D.S. (2005) 'Widening social inequalities in risk for sudden infant death syndrome', *American Journal of Public Health* 95: 1976-81.

Qi, V., Phillips, S. and Hopman, W.M. (2006) 'Determinants of healthy lifestyle and use of preventive screening in Canada', *BMC Public Health* 6: 275.

Raine, R., Hutchings, A. and Black, N. (2003) 'Is publicly funded health care really distributed according to need? The example of cardiac rehabilitation in the UK', *Health Policy* 63: 63-72.

Reading, R., Colver, A., Openshaw, S. and Jarvis, S. (1994) 'Do interventions that improve immunisation uptake also reduce social inequalities in uptake?', *British Medical Journal* 308: 1142-4.

Relton, C.L., Hammal, D.M., Rankin, J. and Parker, L. (2005) 'Folic acid supplementation and social deprivation', *Journal of Public Health Nutrition* 8: 338-40.

Rodgers, E.M. (2003) *Diffusion of innovations*, New York, NY: Simon & Schuster International.

Saxena, S., Eliahoo, J. and Majeed, A. (2002) 'Socioeconomic and ethnic group differences in self reported health status and use of health services by children and young people in England: cross sectional study', *British Medical Journal* 325: 520.

Schellenberg, J.A., Victora, C.G., Mushi, A., de Savigny, D., Schellenberg, D., Mshinda, H. and Bryce, J. (2003) 'Inequities among the very poor: health care for children in rural southern Tanzania', *The Lancet* 361: 561-6.

Scott, A., Shiell, A. and King, M. (1996) 'Is general practitioner decision making associated with patient socio-economic status?', *Social Science and Medicine* 42: 35-46.

Stirling, A.M., Wilson, P. and McConnachie, A. (2001) 'Deprivation, psychological distress, and consultation length in general practice', *British Journal of General Practice* 51: 456-60.

Townsend, J., Roderick, P. and Cooper, J. (1994) 'Cigarette smoking by socioeconomic group, sex, and age: effects of price, income, and health publicity', *British Medical Journal* 309: 923-7.

Townsend, P. and Davidson, N. (1982) *Inequalities in health: The Black Report*, Suffolk: Penguin Books.

Tudor Hart, J. (1971) 'The inverse care law', *The Lancet* 7696: 405-12.

Tugwell, P., Bennett, K.J., Sackett, D.L. and Haynes, R.B. (1985) 'The measurement iterative loop: a framework for the critical appraisal of need, benefits and costs of health interventions', *Journal of Chronic Diseases* 38: 339-51.

Tugwell, P., de Savigny, D., Hawker, G. and Robinson, V. (2006) 'Applying clinical epidemiological methods to health equity: the equity effectiveness loop', *British Medical Journal* 332: 358-61.

Turrell, G., Patterson, C., Oldenburg, B., Gould, T. and Roy, M.A. (2002) 'The socio-economic patterning of survey participation and non-response error in a multilevel study of food purchasing behaviour: areas and individual-level characteristics', *Public Health Nutrition* 6: 181-9.

US Department of Health and Human Services (2000) *Healthy People 2010: Understanding and improving health*, Washington, DC: US Department of Health and Human Services, Government Printing Office.

van Ryn, M. and Fu, S.S. (2003) 'Paved with good intentions: do public health and human service providers contribute to racial/ethnic disparities in health?', *American Journal of Public Health* 93: 248-55.

Victora, C.G., Vaughan, J.P., Barros, F.C., Silva, A.C. and Tomasi, E. (2000) 'Explaining trends in inequalities: evidence from Brazilian child health studies', *The Lancet* 356: 1093-8.

Virtanen, P., Kivimaki, M., Vahtera, J. and Koskenvuo, M. (2006) 'Employment status and differences in the one-year coverage of physician visits: different needs or unequal access to services?', *BMC Health Services Research* 6: 123.

von Elm, E. and Egger, M. (2004) 'The scandal of poor epidemiological research', *British Medical Journal* 329: 868-9.

Wanless, D. (2004) *Securing good health for the whole population*, London: HM Treasury.

Watt, G. (2002) 'The inverse care law today', *The Lancet* 360: 252-4.

Webb, E. (1998) 'Children and the inverse care law', *British Medical Journal* 316: 1588-91.

Wright, C.M. (1997) 'Who comes to be weighed: an exception to the inverse care law', *The Lancet* 350: 642.

SIX

The metaphor of the miner's canary and black–white disparities in health: a review of intergenerational socioeconomic factors and perinatal outcomes

Debbie Barrington

Introduction

In the book *The miner's canary*, Lani Guinier and Gerald Torres (2002) use the metaphor of the miner's canary to describe the predicament of racially marginalised people in the US. Years ago, a canary would be taken into the mines to alert miners to dangerous atmospheric conditions. Since the canary's more sensitive respiratory system would cause it to collapse from any poisonous gases long before humans could be affected, the canary's distress was a signal for an immediate departure from the mine. Guinier and Torres (2002, p 12) write that:

> [T]he miner's canary metaphor helps us to understand why and how race continues to be salient. Racialized communities signal problems with the ways we have structured power and privilege. These pathologies are not located in the canary. Indeed we reject the incrementalist approach that locates complex social and political problems in the individual. Such an approach would solve the problems of the mines by outfitting the canary with a tiny gas mask to withstand the toxic atmosphere.

This powerful metaphor can be extended to racial and ethnic disparities in health where racialised communities share a disproportionate burden of disease. One compelling case concerns the racial disparities in perinatal outcomes. Widening black–white disparity in infant mortality and its critical measures of increased risk, low birth weight (LBW) (born weighing less than 2,500 grams), very LBW (born weighing less than 1,500 grams) and preterm delivery (born at a gestational age less than 37 weeks) continue to be leading public health challenges in the US (US Department of Health and Human Services, 2000). Black-to-white ratios of infant mortality rates were 1.64 in 1950, 2.07 in 1985 and 2.52 in 1999. Natality data for the US also revealed a stable twofold black–white disparity in infant LBW over the past 34 years. In 1970, LBW rates were 13.9% among births to African American women and 6.85% among births to white women. Similarly, in 2004, LBW rates were 13.4% for black infants and 7.1% for white infants (National Center for Health Statistics, 2007). While research on black–white differences in perinatal outcomes has been extensive, isolating the social causes that can eliminate this disparity remains elusive. The metaphor of the miner's canary however, where the 'canaries' symbolise African Americans and the 'miners' represent white people, offers a new framework that can be instructive for research into the black–white disparity in perinatal health.

The social context for many African Americans includes residence within 'toxic mines' or impoverished, segregated neighbourhoods comprised of poor-quality schools and housing, increased levels of environmental contaminants, limited social and health services, poor access to reasonably priced and nutritious food, elevated crime rates, vandalism, high unemployment rates, increased exposure to drugs, alcohol and other poor health behaviours, family disintegration and decreased social support and social ties, whereas most white Americans have limited exposure to these psychosocial stressors within their neighbourhoods (Williams and Collins, 2001). Residence within and characteristics of these segregated disadvantaged environments have been linked to poor perinatal health outcomes. Racial residential segregation has been found to be associated with infant mortality (LaVeist, 1989; Polednak, 1991, 1996). Living within a neighbourhood that has an elevated violent crime rate (Collins and David, 1997), an increased male unemployment rate (Pearl et al, 2001), a high poverty rate (Rauh et al, 2001), low median income (Gould et al, 1989; Collins and David, 1990), decreased homeownership rates (Roberts, 1997) or an increased proportion of families with a female head of household (Gorman, 1999) increases the risk for delivering a LBW infant.

At the individual level, many African Americans as 'canaries' experience the 'toxicity' of low socioeconomic position (SEP), characterised by decreased educational attainment, reduced employment earnings and lower occupational status relative to white people. Black Americans also face interpersonal racial discrimination, confrontation with negative stereotypes as well as internalised racism or identity incorporation of negative stereotypes (Williams, 1999; Jones, 2000). There is longstanding evidence illustrating the damaging effect of low SEP on perinatal and maternal health across the lifecourse for both black and white people (Paneth et al, 1982; Parker et al, 1994; Williams and Collins, 1995). Adjustment for current socioeconomic factors however, does not completely explain the racial differences in infant birth weight, preterm delivery and infant mortality (Kleinman and Kessel, 1987; Miller and Jekel, 1987). Furthermore, the relative racial gap in perinatal outcomes has been found to widen with increasing SEP (McGrady et al, 1992; Schoendorf et al, 1992). Recent perinatal literature has revealed an effect of perceived racial discrimination on the delivery of LBW and very LBW infants, yet most of the effects were too small to account for the racial disparity in perinatal health outcomes (Collins et al, 2000, 2004; Rosenberg et al, 2002; Dole et al, 2003; Mustillo et al, 2004).

The metaphor of the miner's canary, however, points to an underdeveloped area of research that can offer promising insights into eliminating the racial disparities in perinatal health outcomes. The length of time that 'canaries' dwell within the 'mines' as characterised by racial discrimination and low SEP at the individual, familial and neighbourhood levels, as well as the duration that the 'miners' reside external to this toxic atmosphere may have important implications for the reproductive health of both African American and white women. This perspective is akin to a lifecourse epidemiological framework where time and timing are recognised as important for the understanding of causal links between exposures and health outcomes along the lifecourse, across generations and at the population level (Ben-Shlomo and Kuh, 2002; Lynch and Smith, 2005).

Within the US, African Americans have been exposed to these toxic milieux not only for their entire lives, but for generations. As such, intergenerational socioeconomic factors, or socioeconomic conditions, exposures and environments experienced by one generation may be posited to have an impact on the reproductive health of the subsequent generation (Emanuel, 1986). Therefore, research into the effects of intergenerational socioeconomic factors on perinatal health is a promising avenue for investigating the aetiology of the production and reproduction of racial/ethnic disparities in maternal and infant health. This chapter reviews the existing literature that examines the effects of childhood and intergenerational SEP on perinatal outcomes in the US, the UK and Sweden, and discusses how further investigation into these factors may be a fruitful area of exploration for research on racial/ethnic disparities in health.

Intergenerational socioeconomic factors: when canaries are within the mines across generations

Low SEP, irrespective of race, increases the potential for adverse reproductive outcomes during a pregnancy by impeding access to appropriate prenatal care, proper nutrition and good maternal health, by promoting poor health behaviours or maladaptive coping strategies and/or by intensifying physical and emotional stress within the mother (Institute of Medicine, 1985). Nevertheless, as previously described, the relative racial gap in LBW and infant mortality actually widens with increasing SEP. Studies reporting this counterintuitive finding have been cross-sectional, lacking socioeconomic information over the lifecourse, yet how long a black mother has held her current SEP at the individual, familial and neighbourhood level must be evaluated. Most African American families of high SEP are 'newly arrived', able to obtain middle-class status only after the civil rights legislations in the 1960s attempted to reverse centuries of social and economic deprivation resulting from governmental and culturally sanctioned racism (Collins, 1997). As a result, middle-class black people do not have the multigenerational lifestyle, educational, economic or class stability that typifies a middle-class white family (Foster et al, 1993). Furthermore, SEP is an intergenerational in addition to an intragenerational phenomenon where parental SEP influences childhood well-being, educational achievement and later adult socioeconomic attainment and health (House and Williams, 2000). Hence, factors operating long antecedent to pregnancy, within a mother's early childhood or even intergenerational in nature, may be possible explanations for the persistent perinatal health disadvantage among black infants relative to white infants irrespective of current SEP (Emanuel et al, 1989; Foster, 1997).

Moreover, recent scientific evidence has revealed that the maternal environment during pregnancy may have health implications not only for foetal development in utero, but also for the child's development over the lifecourse into adulthood. This direction of research has been sparked by the 'Barker hypothesis' or 'foetal programming hypothesis', which posits that foetal undernourishment in middle or late gestation of pregnancy not only results in disproportionate foetal growth and infant LBW, but also programmes later cardiovascular disease in adulthood (Barker, 1993, 1994). Since the Barker hypothesis has been proposed, numerous studies have found links between infant LBW and adult hypertension, coronary heart disease (Law and Barker, 1994; Klebanoff et al, 1999) and Type 2 diabetes (Law, 1996; Rich-Edwards et al, 1999).

Most importantly, evidence from epidemiological studies supports the foetal programming of reproductive health outcomes. A number of investigations have uncovered a positive independent association between maternal birth weight and infant LBW (Little, 1987; Emanuel et al, 1992; Coutinho et al, 1997; Skjaerven et al, 1997; Collins et al, 2003). Through foetal undernourishment and increased cortisol levels, maternal stress during pregnancy has been postulated as a major factor in the foetal programming of birth outcomes within the subsequent generation (Klebanoff and Yip, 1987; Leff et al, 1992). Given that chronic maternal stress ultimately traces back to a mother's social circumstances, including her relative SEP in society, investigations into the influence of the social context surrounding a mother's pregnancy within one generation on the perinatal outcome of the next generation can be informative research endeavours.

In addition to the foetal programming or latency model, which theorises that exposures at critical in utero periods may have longlasting effects on reproductive health, under a cumulative burden pathway model (Power and Hertzman, 1997) common social and environmental factors between generations are postulated to explain the positive correlations of birth weight across the generations (Magnus et al, 1993; Sanderson et al, 1995). African American women may experience increased maternal stress relative to white women through a greater cumulative exposure of adverse societal conditions resulting from low SEP and experiences of racial discrimination along the lifecourse. Moreover, black Americans may have a greater vulnerability to stress exposure as a consequence of in utero programming of the HPA-axis (Hogue et al, 2001; Matthews, 2002; Lu and Halfon, 2003). This increased vulnerability to stress is akin to the more sensitive respiratory system of the 'canaries' relative to the 'miners'. Therefore, through a critical period mechanism and/or an accumulation of risk lifecourse model, intergenerational SEP characterised by those socioeconomic conditions, exposures and environments experienced by one generation that relate to the health, growth and development of the next generation may be an important contributor to the poorer perinatal health outcomes replicated across time among the ill-fated 'canaries' relative to the 'miners'.

The effects of childhood and intergenerational socioeconomic factors on infant birth outcomes

The epidemiological literature is limited in regards to studies that have examined the influence of SEP on the perinatal outcomes of subsequent generations, yet the proposition to investigate the reproductive health impact of either childhood or intergenerational SEP is not a novel one. As early as the 1930s, the term 'generational mortalities' appeared in the scientific literature to describe the view that the health and reproductive health of an individual is determined by their social environment from birth through childhood (Kermack et al, 1934). Later, in the 1950s, the notion of generational mortalities re-emerged within the scientific literature to explain the consistent stepwise rates of infant mortality at decreasing levels of social class within Britain between 1911 and 1950 (Morris and Heady, 1955). This hypothesis sparked a new direction of empirical research, which began to analyse the effects of childhood SEP, and most notably, intergenerational SEP on perinatal outcomes.

Baird and Illsley (1953) used a composite measure of SEP comprised of the social class of both a woman's husband and her father when examining the effects of social class on perinatal health outcomes within the UK. According to the authors, the social class of a woman's husband reflected the social conditions during her pregnancy and marriage, while the main occupation of a woman's father during her school years represented the social conditions of her upbringing. Women who were in the highest social classes during their childhood and marriage had the lowest rate of premature delivery. Those who experienced substantial downward social class mobility, spending their childhood within the highest social class, but marrying a husband in the lowest social class, had the highest rate of premature delivery. Finally, those women who experienced upward social class mobility at marriage had lower rates of premature delivery as compared to those who experienced no mobility (Illsley, 1955; Baird, 1962).

Also during the 1950s, Drillien (1957) reported that within the UK the social class of a mother's father was more closely correlated with the incidence of infant LBW and preterm delivery than the social class of a mother's husband. She also found an association between these perinatal outcomes and unemployment of the infant's grandfather when the mother was a child. Furthermore, decades after his original findings, later work by Baird (1974, 1980) examined intergenerational socioeconomic effects on perinatal outcomes and showed that the socioeconomic conditions at the time of a mother's birth was an important factor influencing the incidence of LBW and perinatal mortality.

Joffe's (1989) analyses of the British National Child Development Study (NCDS) showed that having a higher social class at birth as determined by the grandfather's occupation at the mother's birth had a protective effect on infant LBW. Moreover, Emanuel et al (1992) observed within the NCDS that a grandfather's social class, characterised as having a manual as compared to a non-manual occupation at the mother's birth, decreased infant birth weight. Batty et al (2005) showed within the Aberdeen cohort study a similar decrease in infant birth weight among Scottish mothers who were born to fathers having a manual as compared to a non-manual occupation. Selling et al (2006) reported that the grandmother's educational level at the time of giving birth to the mother was independently associated with preterm birth among two generations of women residing in Sweden even after adjustment for the mother's current SEP, smoking habits and BMI. Finally, Spencer (2004) reported that both intergenerational and early childhood factors accounted for 10.3 grams of the birth weight disparity between social classes in Britain.

The first studies examining the effects of childhood SEP on perinatal outcomes among black women within the US yielded slightly different results than those findings reported by the European studies. Udry et al (1970) examined the relationship between childhood SEP and birth outcomes among married black women in the District of Columbia from 1965 to 1966. They could not show that those women from lower social class backgrounds, as characterised by the occupation of the head of the household when the mother was 10-14 years of age, had higher LBW rates than those women from middle-class backgrounds irrespective of present class status as determined by the husband's occupation. African American women who were upwardly mobile, moving from lower to middle class, had a lower rate of infant LBW than those who stayed within a lower class from childhood to adulthood. Those black women who were downwardly mobile, moving from the middle class in childhood to a lower class as adults, had a higher rate of infant LBW than those who remained within the middle class throughout their lifecourse. However, those black women who were in the middle class when they were children as well as when they were adults had similar rates of infant LBW relative to those who remained in the lower class from childhood through adulthood.

Valanis (Valanis, 1979; Valanis and Rush, 1979) studied black female participants in a randomised prenatal nutritional supplementation trial in New York City from 1971 to 1973 who had originated from either New York City, the southern region of the US or foreign countries within South America, Africa and the Caribbean. Her study revealed an association between childhood SEP and infant birth weight. Yet, the positive linear relationship with infant birth weight and childhood social status as defined by either the maternal or the paternal occupation of the gravida's parents during childhood was only observed among foreign-born black women and not among native-born black women. Selection due to missing data, however, may explain the null association between childhood SEP and infant birth weight among native-born black women, for only 6% of foreign-born black women did not know their father's occupation during their childhood as compared to 42% of black mothers from New York City and 29% of black women from the South.

Later empirical investigations that focused on the effects of intergenerational SEP on perinatal outcomes among both black and white people in the US demonstrated similar associations to those reported by the European studies. Hackman et al (1983) found that the grandmother's marital status at the time of the mother's birth had a significant correlation with infant birth weight. Foster et al (2000), comparing births from two generations of college-educated US black and white women, found that there was a narrowing of the racial differential in LBW due to the sustained high SEP in the African American population. Berg et al (2001) reported that among Georgian white people, maternal grandfathers of normal birth-weight infants were twice as likely to have graduated from college compared to maternal grandfathers of very LBW infants. Poerkson and Petitti (1991) found within their study of African American women in California that logistic models that included educational mobility in addition to current maternal socioeconomic circumstances – that is, maternal education, income, occupation and marital status – explained more variation in infant LBW, as compared to models that incorporated only the current SEP of the mother.

Furthermore, Conley and Bennett (2001) reported an interaction between maternal LBW and poverty where there was an effect of maternal LBW on infant LBW only among those mothers who were born into poverty. Astone et al (2007) showed that the grandmother's household income and education in addition to maternal education were found to be positively and significantly associated with infant birth weight. Finally, Currie and Moretti (2007) found that household income at the time of a mother's birth was associated with her infant's LBW status. They also uncovered an interaction between maternal LBW and poverty in the production of infant LBW where the intergenerational transmission of LBW was stronger for mothers who were poor as compared to those who were not poor.

Discussion

In this chapter the existing literature on the role of childhood and intergenerational SEP in the production of perinatal health outcomes has been reviewed. Under the framework specified by the metaphor of the miner's canary, the length of time that black women reside within a toxic social environment across the lifecourse, in utero through the reproductive period, is an important contributor to black people's poorer perinatal health relative to white people. Extant research examining the effect of intergenerational SEP on perinatal health outcomes among Europeans, African Americans and European Americans have found evidence of an independent effect of the socioeconomic context surrounding the pregnancy of one generation on the perinatal outcomes of the subsequent generation. Furthermore, recent studies have found that the intergenerational transmission of poor perinatal outcomes interacts with SEP. The reproduction of infant LBW across the generations is stronger among those mothers who are born into social conditions at the lower end than at the upper end of the socioeconomic spectrum. These findings have both methodological and political implications for racial/ ethnic disparities research.

The miner's canary framework and its emphasis on the importance of intergenerational socioeconomic factors in the production and reproduction of racial/ethnic disparities in perinatal health reveal several methodological challenges in health disparities research that essentially compares 'miners' with 'canaries'. Class structure or SEP gives race its meaning in the US, as colour symbolises the inequality of power relations and the ownership of property and resources (Mullings, 1997). Yet, there may be threats to the validity of a study when socioeconomic factors are controlled for to determine whether an observed racial disparity can be explained by differences in social class (Krieger et al, 1993; Kaufman et al, 1997; Kaufman and Cooper, 2001).

First, an inaccurate conceptualisation of SEP that uses as a proxy a one-dimensional measure such as educational level can produce residual confounding and biased racial effects, for the necessary assumption of comparability within each category of this social class indicator is often violated. For example, the economic return in terms of salary, benefits, occupation, wealth and/or residence in an affluent neighbourhood for the same level of education is lower among African Americans than for white people (Krieger et al, 1997; Williams, 2002).

Second, the relationship between a particular socioeconomic indicator and a specific reproductive health outcome may differ markedly between African American and white women (Parker et al, 1994; Braveman et al, 2001), that is, the social factors may operate through different mechanisms for the 'miners' and the 'canaries'.

Third, the sampled racial groups under study may lack sufficient overlap in the socioeconomic indicators since most 'canaries' reside within the toxic mines while most 'miners' are located outside them. This prohibits ordinary statistical methods such as multivariable logistic regression to legitimately perform adjustment for confounding due to SEP.

Finally, as suggested by this review, analysing only current socioeconomic factors surrounding a pregnancy will further reduce comparability between racial groups, for black and white people have distinctly different class backgrounds. Since additional socioeconomic information along a woman's lifecourse, such as childhood SEP, as well as socioeconomic information across the generations, that is, intergenerational SEP, have been found to be related to maternal and infant health, the exclusion of these supplementary, but significant socioeconomic factors will serve to further amplify residual confounding and biased racial effects.

The framework of the miner's canary with its focus on the importance of both in utero and cumulative socioeconomic exposures along the lifecourse also provides key policy and research recommendations for eliminating the racial disparities in perinatal outcomes. Under the tenets of this metaphor, if the health of the 'canaries' is improved, the health for all Americans is also enhanced. Therefore, the optimal policy recommendation would be to eradicate the 'toxicity' or more specifically the poverty that exists within the mines. As of 2002, 13% of white children and 32% of black children resided within impoverished families in the US (National Center for Health Statistics, 2004). As suggested by this review, female children living within a social context of poverty will not only be more likely to have been born with LBW, but they will also have an increased probability of transmitting this poor perinatal outcome to the next generation. Hence, the twofold risk of poverty among African American relative to white children is correlated with both the contemporary twofold disparity in infant LBW as well as the future reproduction of that disparity within the subsequent generation.

Accordingly, policies that work within the current generation to eliminate childhood poverty and maternal deprivation during pregnancy must extend their evaluation of these interventions into the next generation. Continued epidemiological research into the effects of childhood and intergenerational SEP on maternal and infant health outcomes will also remain informative for understanding and eventually eliminating the racial/ethnic disparities in perinatal health outcomes. Additional longitudinal studies similar to the Millennium Cohort Study initiated in 2001 in the UK (Hansen, 2003) are needed to link exposures to risk and protective factors at multiple levels over the lifecourse and across generations. These studies will provide knowledge of the mechanisms of risk that can be severed to enhance maternal and infant health, but as the miner's canary framework suggests, this level of intervention can only serve to outfit the 'canaries' with tiny gas masks. The greater purpose for this longitudinal research, however, is to provide additional evidence necessary for eradicating the toxicity within the mines. This will serve to improve maternal and infant health for all, for once the 'miners' enter the mines they too will be affected by the toxic atmosphere just like the 'canaries'.

References

Astone, N.M., Misra, D.P. and Johnson, C. (2007) 'The effect of maternal socioeconomic status on infant birthweight', *Paediatric and Perinatal Epidemiology* 21: 310-18.

Baird, D. (1962) 'Environmental and obstetrical factors in prematurity, with special reference to experience in Aberdeen', *Bulletin of the World Health Organization* 26: 291-5.

Baird, D. (1974) 'The epidemiology of low birth weight; changes in incidence in Aberdeen, 1948–72', *Journal of Biosocial Science* 6: 323-41.

Baird, D. (1980) 'Environment and Reproduction', *British Journal of Obstetrics and Gynaecology* 87: 1057-67.

Baird, D. and Illsley, R. (1953) 'Environment and childbearing', *Proceedings of the Royal Society of Medicine* 46: 53-9.

Barker, D.J. (1993) 'The intrauterine origins of cardiovascular disease', *Acta Paediatrica Supplement 82* (Suppl 391): 93-9; discussion 100.

Barker, D.J. (1994) 'Maternal and fetal origins of coronary heart disease', *Journal of the Royal College of Physicians* 28: 544–51.

Batty, G.D., Lawlor, D.A., Macintyre, S., Clark, H. and Leon, D.A. (2005) 'Accuracy of adults' recall of childhood social class: findings from the Aberdeen Children of the 1950s Study', *Journal of Epidemiology and Community Health* 59: 898–903.

Ben-Shlomo, Y. and Kuh, D. (2002) 'A life course approach to chronic disease epidemiology: conceptual models, empirical challenges and interdisciplinary perspectives', *International Journal of Epidemiology* 31: 285–93.

Berg, C.J., Wilcox, L.S. and d'Almada, P.J. (2001) 'The prevalence of socioeconomic and behavioral characteristics and their impact on very low birth weight in black and white infants in Georgia', *Maternal and Child Health Journal* 5: 75–84.

Braveman, P., Cubbin, C., Marchi, K., Egerter, S. and Chavez, G. (2001) 'Measuring socioeconomic status/position in studies of racial/ethnic disparities: maternal and infant health', *Public Health Reports* 116: 449–63.

Collins, J.W., Jr, and David, R.J. (1990) 'The differential effect of traditional risk-factors on infant birth-weight among Blacks and Whites in Chicago', *American Journal of Public Health* 80: 679–81.

Collins, J.W., Jr, and David, R.J. (1997) 'Urban violence and African-American pregnancy outcome: an ecologic study', *Ethnicity and Disease* 7:184–90.

Collins, J.W., Jr, David, R.J., Handler, A., Wall, S. and Andes, S. (2004) 'Very low birthweight in African American infants: the role of maternal exposure to interpersonal racial discrimination', *American Journal of Public Health* 94: 2132–8.

Collins, J.W., Jr, David, R.J., Prachand, N.G. and Pierce, M.L. (2003) 'Low birth weight across generations', *Maternal and Child Health Journal* 7: 229–37.

Collins, J.W., Jr, David, R.J., Symons, R., Handler, A., Wall, S.N. and Dwyer, L. (2000) 'Low-income African-American mothers' perception of exposure to racial discrimination and infant birth weight', *Epidemiology* 11: 337–9.

Collins, S.M. (1997) *Black corporate executives: The making and breaking of a black middle class*, Philadelphia: Temple University Press.

Conley, D. and Bennett, N.G. (2001) 'Birth weight and income: interactions across generations', *Journal of Health and Social Behaviours* 42: 450–65.

Coutinho, R., David, R.J. and Collins, J.W., Jr (1997) 'Relation of parental birth weights to infant birth weight among African Americans and Whites in Illinois: a transgenerational study', *American Journal of Epidemiology* 146: 804–9.

Currie, J. and Moretti, E. (2007) 'Biology as destiny? Short and long-run determinants of intergenerational transmission of birth weight', *Journal of Labour Economics* 25: 231–63.

Dole, N., Savitz, D.A., Hertz-Picciotto, I., Siega-Riz, A.M., McMahon, M.J. and Buekens, P. (2003) 'Maternal stress and preterm birth', *American Journal of Epidemiology* 157: 14–24.

Drillien, C.M. (1957) 'The social and economic factors affecting the incidence of premature birth. I. Premature births without complications of pregnancy', *The Journal of Obstetrics and Gynaecology of the British Empire* 64: 161–84.

Emanuel, I. (1986) 'Maternal health during childhood and later reproductive performance', *Annals of the New York Academy of Sciences* 477: 27-39.

Emanuel, I., Filakti, H., Alberman, E. and Evans, S.J. (1992) 'Intergenerational studies of human birthweight from the 1958 birth cohort. 1. Evidence for a multigenerational effect', *British Journal of Obstetrics and Gynaecology* 99: 67-74.

Emanuel, I., Hale, C.B. and Berg C.J. (1989) 'Poor birth outcomes of American Black Women: an alternative explanation', *Journal of Public Health Policy* 10: 299-308.

Foster, H.W., Jr (1997) 'The enigma of low birth weight and race', *The New England Journal of Medicine* 337: 1232-3.

Foster, H.W., Jr, Thomas, D.J., Semenya, K.A. and Thomas J. (1993) 'Low birthweight in African Americans: does intergenerational well-being improve outcome?', *Journal of the National Medical Association* 85: 516-20.

Foster, H.W., Wu, L., Bracken, M.B., Semenya, K., Thomas, J. and Thomas, J. (2000) 'Intergenerational effects of high socioeconomic status on low birthweight and preterm birth in African Americans', *Journal of the National Medical Association* 92: 213-21.

Gorman, B.K. (1999) 'Racial and ethnic variation in low birthweight in the United States: individual and contextual determinants', *Health & Place* 5: 195-207.

Gould, J.B., Davey, B. and LeRoy, S. (1989) 'Socioeconomic differentials and neonatal mortality: racial comparison of California singletons', *Pediatrics* 83: 181-6.

Guiner, L. and Torres, G. (2002) *The miner's canary: Enlisting race, resisting power, transforming democracy*, Cambridge, MA: Harvard University Press.

Hackman, E., Emanuel, I., van Belle, G. and Daling, J. (1983) 'Maternal birth weight and subsequent pregnancy outcome', *JAMA* 250: 2016-19.

Hansen, K. (ed) (2003) *Millennium cohort study: First and second surveys*, London: Institute of Education, University of London.

Hogue, C.J., Hoffman, S. and Hatch, M.C. (2001) 'Stress and preterm delivery: a conceptual framework', *Paediatric and Perinatal Epidemiology* 15(Suppl 2): 30-40.

House, J.R. and Williams, D.R. (2000) 'Understanding and reducing socioeconomic and racial/ethnic disparities in health', in B.D. Smedley and S.L. Syme (eds) *Promoting health intervention strategies from social and behavioral research*, Washington, DC: National Academy Press: 81-124.

Institute of Medicine Division of Health Promotion and Disease Prevention Committee to Study the Prevention of Low Birthweight (1985) *Preventing low birth-weight*, Washington, DC: National Academy Press.

Illsley, R. (1955) 'Social class selection and class differences in relation to stillbirths and infant deaths', *British Medical Journal* 1520-4.

Joffe, M. (1989) 'Social inequalities in low birth-weight: timing of effects and selective mobility', *Social Science & Medicine* 28: 613-19.

Jones, C.P. (2000) 'Levels of racism: a theoretic framework and a gardener's tale', *American Journal of Public Health* 90: 1212-5.

Kaufman, J.S. and Cooper, R.S. (2001) 'Commentary: considerations for use of racial/ethnic classification in etiologic research', *American Journal of Epidemiology* 154: 291-8.

Kaufman, J.S., Cooper, R.S. and McGee, D. L. (1997) 'Socioeconomic status and health in Blacks and Whites: the problem of residual confounding and the resiliency of race', *Epidemiology* 8: 621-8.

Kermack, W.O., McKendrick, A.G. and McKinlay, P.L. (1934) 'Death rates in Great Britain and Sweden: some general regularities and their significance', *Lancet* 31: 698-703.

Klebanoff, M.A. and Yip, R. (1987) 'Influence of maternal birth weight on rate of fetal growth and duration of gestation', *The Journal of Pediatrics* 111: 287-92.

Klebanoff, M.A., Secher, N.J., Mednick, B. R. and Schulsinger, .C. (1999) 'Maternal size at birth and the development of hypertension during pregnancy: a test of the Barker hypothesis', *Archives of Internal Medicine* 159: 1607-12.

Kleinman, J.C. and Kessel, S.S. (1987) 'Racial differences in low birth weight. trends and risk factors', *New England Journal of Medicine* 317: 749-53.

Krieger, N., Rowley, D.L., Herman, A.A., Avery, B. and Phillips, M.T. (1993) 'Racism, sexism, and social class: implications for studies of health, disease, and well-being', *American Journal of Preventive Medicine* 9: 82-122.

Krieger, N., Williams, D.R. and Moss, N.E. (1997) 'Measuring social class in US public health research: concepts, methodologies, and guidelines', *Annual Review of Public Health* 18: 341-78.

LaVeist, T. A. (1989) 'Linking residential segregation to the infant-mortality race disparity in United States cities', *Sociology and Social Research* 73: 90-4.

Law, C.M. (1996) 'Fetal and infant influences on non-insulin-dependent diabetes mellitus (NIDDM)', *Diabetic Medicine* 13: S49-S52.

Law, C.M. and Barker, D. J. (1994) 'Fetal influences on blood pressure', *Journal of Hypertension* 12: 1329-32.

Leff, M., Orleans, M., Haverkamp, A.D., Baron, A.E., Alderman, B.W. and Freedman, W. L. (1992) 'The association of maternal low birthweight and infant low birthweight in a racially mixed population', *Paediatric and Perinatal Epidemiology* 6: 51-61.

Little, R.E. (1987) 'Mother's and father's birthweight as predictors of infant birthweight', *Paediatric and Perinatal Epidemiology* 1: 19-31.

Lu, M.C. and Halfon, N. (2003) 'Racial and ethnic disparities in birth outcomes: a life-course perspective', *Maternal and Child Health Journal* 7: 13-30.

Lynch, J., and Smith, G.D. (2005) 'A life course approach to chronic disease epidemiology', *Annual Review of Public Health* 26: 1-35.

Magnus, P., Bakketeig, L.S. and Skjaerven, R. (1993) 'Correlations of birth weight and gestational age across generations', *Annals of Human Biology* 20: 231-8.

Matthews, S.G. (2002) 'Early programming of the hypothalamo-pituitary-adrenal axis', *Trends in Endocrinology and Metabolism* 13: 373-80.

McGrady, G.A., Sung, J. F., Rowley, D.L. and Hogue, C.J. (1992) 'Preterm delivery and low birth weight among first-born infants of black and white college graduates', *American Journal of Epidemiology* 136: 266-76.

Miller, H.C. and Jekel, J.F. (1987) 'The effect of race on the incidence of low birth weight: persistence of effect after controlling for socioeconomic, educational, marital, and risk status', *Yale Journal of Biology and Medicine* 60: 221-32.

Morris, J.N. and Heady, J.A. (1955) 'V. Mortality in relation to the father's occupation; 1911–1950', *Lancet* 268: 554-60.

Mullings, L. (1997) *On our own terms: Race, class, and gender in the lives of African American women*, New York: Routledge.

Mustillo, S., Krieger, N., Gunderson, E.P., Sidney, S., McCreath, H. and Kiefe, C.I. (2004) 'Self-reported experiences of racial discrimination and black–white differences in preterm and low-birthweight deliveries: the CARDIA study', *American Journal of Public Health* 94: 2125-31.

National Center for Health Statistics. (2007) *Health, United States, 2007 with chartbook on trends in the health of Americans*, Hyattsville, MD: Government Printing Office.

Paneth, N., Wallenstein, S., Kiely, J.L. and Susser, M. (1982) 'Social class indicators and mortality in low birth weight infants', *American Journal of Epidemiology* 116: 364-75.

Parker, J.D., Schoendorf, K.C. and Kiely, J.L. (1994) 'Associations between measures of socioeconomic status and low birth weight, small for gestational age, and premature delivery in the United States', *Annals of Epidemiology* 4: 271-8.

Pearl, M., Braveman, P. and Abrams, B. (2001) 'The relationship of neighborhood socioeconomic characteristics to birthweight among 5 ethnic groups in California', *American Journal of Public Health* 91: 1808-14.

Poerksen, A. and Petitti, D.B. (1991) 'Employment and low birth weight in black women', *Social Science and Medicine* 33: 1281-6.

Polednak, A.P. (1991) 'Black–White differences in infant-mortality in 38 standard metropolitan statistical areas', *American Journal of Public Health* 81: 1480-82.

Polednak, A.P. (1996) 'Trends in US urban black infant mortality, by degree of residential segregation', *American Journal of Public Health* 86: 723-26.

Power, C. and Hertzman, C. (1997) 'Social and biological pathways linking early life and adult disease', *British Medical Bulletin* 53: 210-21.

Rauh, V.A., Andrews, H.F. and Garfinkel, R.S. (2001) 'The contribution of maternal age to racial disparities in birthweight: a multilevel perspective', *American Journal of Public Health* 91: 1815-24.

Rich-Edwards, J.W., Colditz, G.A., Stampfer, M.J., Willett, W.C., Gillman, M.W., Hennekens, C.H., Speizer, F.E. and Manson, J.E. (1999) 'Birthweight and the risk for type 2 diabetes mellitus in adult women', *Annals of Internal Medicine* 130: 278-84.

Roberts, E.M. (1997) 'Neighborhood social environments and the distribution of low birthweight in Chicago', *American Journal of Public Health* 87: 597-603.

Rosenberg, L., Palmer, J.R., Wise, L.A., Horton, N.J. and Corwin, M.J. (2002) 'Perceptions of racial discrimination and the risk of preterm birth', *Epidemiology* 13: 646-52.

Sanderson, M., Emanuel, I. and Holt, V.L. (1995) 'The intergenerational relationship between mother's birthweight, infant birthweight and infant mortality in black and white mothers', *Paediatric and Perinatal Epidemiology* 9: 391-405.

Schoendorf, K.C., Hogue, C.J., Kleinman, J.C. and Rowley, D. (1992) 'Mortality among infants of black as compared with white college-educated parents', *The New England Journal of Medicine* 326: 1522-6.

Selling, K.E., Carstensen, J., Finnstrom, O. and Sydsjo, G. (2006) 'Intergenerational effects of preterm birth and reduced intrauterine growth: a population-based study of Swedish mother-offspring pairs', *BJOG: An International Journal of Obstetrics and Gynaeocology* 113: 430-40.

Skjaerven, R., Wilcox, A.J., Oyen, N. and Magnus, P. (1997) 'Mothers' birth weight and survival of their offspring: population based study', *British Medical Journal* 314: 1376-80.

Spencer, N. (2004) 'Accounting for the social disparity in birth weight: results from an intergenerational cohort', *Journal of Epidemiology and Community Health* 58: 418-9.

Udry, J.R., Morris, N.M., Bauman, K.E. and Chase, C.L. (1970) 'Social class, social mobility, and prematurity: a test of the childhood environment hypothesis for Negro women', *Journal of Health and Social Behavior* 11: 190-5.

US Department of Health and Human Services (2000) *Healthy people 2010: Understanding and improving health*, Washington, DC: US Government Printing Office.

Valanis, B.M. (1979) 'Relative contributions of maternal social and biological characteristics to birth weight and gestation among mothers of different childhood socioeconomic status', *Social Biology* 26: 211-25.

Valanis, B.M., and Rush, D. (1979) 'A partial explanation of superior birth weights among foreign-born women', *Social Biology* 26: 198-210.

Williams, D.R. (1999) 'Race, socioeconomic status, and health. the added effects of racism and discrimination', *Annals of the New York Academy of Sciences* 896: 173-88.

Williams, D.R. (2002) 'Racial/ethnic variations in women's health: the social embeddedness of health', *American Journal of Public Health* 92: 588-97.

Williams, D.R., and Collins, C. (1995) 'US socioeconomic and racial differences in health: patterns and explanations', *Annual Review of Sociology* 21: 349-86.

Williams, D.R. and Collins, C. (2001) 'Racial residential segregation: a fundamental cause of racial disparities in health', *Public Health Reports* 116: 404-16.

SEVEN

From adversary to ally: the evolution of non-governmental organisations in the context of health reform in Santiago and Montevideo

Javier Pereira Bruno and Ronald Angel

Introduction

The non-governmental organisation (NGO), which traces the beginning of its modern mission to the need to rebuild a Europe ravaged by the Second World War, represents an organisational form that is rapidly evolving in response to complex global, national and local forces, and that at the same time is redefining the role of the state and of civil society in the provision of social services. Despite the relatively recent global and large-scale proliferation of the NGO phenomenon, they have existed for centuries. Their founding philosophy is perhaps best embodied in the religious requirement that the pious believer practise good works and minister to the poor. In more recent manifestations their role has often been to reaffirm the domain of civil society in opposition to repressive states. Today, neither the simple philosophy of good works nor the role of opposition adequately summarises the purpose or function of the large-scale, professionalised and internationally funded organisations that sponsor more local activities. Nor do they adequately characterise the function of local NGOs that find their original role as adversaries of repressive governments changing more towards that of allies of national, regional and municipal administrations in providing social services to indigent and vulnerable populations.

During the last few decades, a growing body of theoretical and empirical work underscores the growing importance of the non-governmental sector in areas such as human rights, sustainable development, the environment, education and health. Much of this work is based on case studies and deals with the nature of the relationship between what have been characterised as 'northern' NGOs – the large multinational organisations such as Oxfam International, CARE, Human Rights Watch and hundreds of others that have their headquarters in Europe or the US and that funnel money to 'southern' NGOs that are in direct contact with the target populations – and these southern NGOs (Fowler, 1988; Clark, 1991; Pearce, 1993; Renshaw, 1994; Benett and Gibbs, 1996). Much work also deals with the role of governmental entities such as the International Agency for International Development (USAID) and the United Nations in defining the mission of local NGOs.

One recent research initiative attempts to catalogue and categorise these organisations for the purpose of international comparison (Salamon and Anheier, 1994, 1998, 1999). Despite this body of research, though, the NGO phenomenon remains poorly understood, especially in terms of the ways in which individual organisations have evolved in response to global forces. Meanwhile, the growth in the number of NGOs has accelerated in all nations, a fact that has led some observers to characterise the phenomenon as the internationalisation of civil society and to view NGOs themselves as the vehicles of a global culture (Meyer and Hannan, 1979; Thomas et al, 1987; Boli and Thomas, 1999). The pervasiveness of the phenomenon calls for new theoretical understandings as well as empirical data. Somewhere between the level of the case study and the level of global culture and grand theory lies a middle ground in which the study of individual organisations can be related to larger national, regional and global changes.

In this chapter we draw on newly collected qualitative data concerning the role of specific NGOs in the healthcare sectors of two Latin American countries – Chile and Uruguay – in order to develop a theoretical model of factors that determine the extent of state/NGO cooperation or conflict in the health sector. We focus on these two Southern Cone countries because of their relatively advanced public healthcare systems, and because of the fact that specific state policies result in different opportunities for NGOs in the healthcare sectors of each. In both countries, resistance to military dictatorships during the 1970s and 1980s mobilised organisations that define civil society, of which the NGO represented a new and powerful expression. In both countries, NGOs have served as public venues for the mobilisation of resistance to repressive power, while at the same time reaching out to poor communities that are underserved by the ascendant neoliberal economic policies.

Observers of this period attribute the emergence of the new civil society that includes an expanded role for NGOs to the convergence of the interests and strategies of three sets of actors. These include:

- highly educated middle-class professionals and technicians who were influenced by the social and political militancy of the late 1960s and 1970s;
- the international community, influenced to a large extent by political exiles, which furthered the process of democratisation;
- social activists and community leaders who were interested in creating a new social movement to further democratic reforms and improve the lot of those who had been marginalised by earlier regimes (De la Maza and Ochsenius, 2001).

Since the 1970s, both countries have experienced political and administrative decentralisation, but to different degrees, especially in terms of social services, and both have participated to different degrees in the region's economic liberalisation. While Chile transferred primary healthcare and education to municipal governments in the early years of the Pinochet regime, Uruguay remained closer to its traditional, more centralised, system of social welfare services. Perhaps most importantly, both countries have experienced the restoration of democracy following a period of dictatorship that concluded in 1985 in Uruguay and 1991 in Chile. As a result of these changes, the NGO sector finds its role evolving from that of an adversary of repressive regimes to that of an ally of the state, or at least a complementary organisational form, in the provision of services to the poor.

The Chilean and Uruguayan healthcare systems

We focus on the healthcare sector because of the fact that, like education, medical care is a common necessity that determines national, as well as individual, productivity. Modern medical care is by its very nature highly technical, bureaucratised and expensive. National governments face the growing challenge of providing basic care to all citizens at the same time that they are forced to deal with a period of protracted fiscal austerity. The health sector, then, provides a unique arena in which to examine the evolving relationship between the state and NGOs in providing basic social services.

Like the vast majority of nations, Chile and Uruguay have witnessed an increasing diversity of organisational and administrative arrangements related to healthcare that involve the public, private and non-profit sectors. Much of this change results from the unique nature of the healthcare sector. Healthcare cannot be extensively privatised since large segments of the population cannot afford to pay for services, nor can it be entirely funded by governments with limited resources, and especially in an era of neoliberalisation that seeks to maximise the role of the market. Our questions relate to how the healthcare functions of NGOs are defined and by whom, how these organisations fund their healthcare operations and how they coordinate their efforts with government entities and other NGOs. Our study is primarily qualitative and draws on in-depth interviews in both countries with organisations that provide a wide range of health-related services. It in no way represents an exhaustive census of such organisations.

Currently, little is known of the impact or effectiveness of NGOs in general (Edwards and Hulme, 1996) or of their contribution to healthcare in particular (UNAIDS, 2002; DeJong, 2003). An assessment of effectiveness must begin with a more complete understanding of the functions these organisations play within the broader healthcare sector. In most nations, current debates concerning healthcare financing and delivery remain focused on the role of the state as the principal financer and provider of healthcare. In most developed nations, populations have come to expect government-sponsored care, and no nation is moving in the direction of large-scale privatisation. Even in the US, perhaps the most market-based healthcare system in the world, the introduction of Medicaid and Medicare has resulted in an increasing role of government in the financing of healthcare (Twombly, 2001; Gais et al, 2003). In Latin America, social service reform has focused on a greater emphasis on municipal control of service delivery (Prud'Homme, 1995; Fox and Aranda, 1996; Mesa-Lago and Cruz-Saco, 1999; Willis et al, 1999). In these debates the potential role of NGOs in healthcare delivery remains largely ignored. Yet much preventive and palliative care and certainly much healthcare education including that related to sexual and reproductive health is not highly technical and much of it may well be effectively delivered in the community.

Healthcare sector reform in Chile and Uruguay

Chilean neoliberal healthcare reforms began in 1979 under Pinochet and consisted of four major initiatives. These included:

- the creation of private for-profit healthcare organisations formally known as *Instituciones de Salud Previsional* (ISAPREs);
- the segmentation of the public sector financed primarily by the *Fondo Nacional de Salud* (FONASA), and the restriction of state-financed health services to those areas with insufficient capacity or a lack of private sector interest;
- the decentralisation of health services through the creation of regional administrative and financial authorities;
- the municipalisation of primary healthcare (Miranda, 1994).

Although governmental expenditures for health increased by nearly 240% during the 1990s, large segments of the population remain dissatisfied with the care they receive. Per capita expenditures have increased more rapidly for those enrolled in the ISAPREs than for those who rely on public services. Even though some of the ISAPREs are registered as non-profit organisations, like most for-profit health insurance plans they cream off those with higher incomes and the most favourable health risk profiles, leaving the poor and the sick to the public system. Because of differences in local revenue-generation capacities the municipalisation of primary healthcare has further increased disparities in health expenditures (Miranda, 1994). In order to address these problems, in 2004 the Lagos administration introduced a new wave of reforms designed to implement a universal health plan that assures at least a minimum package of healthcare for every Chilean citizen. *Plan AUGE (Acceso Universal con Garantías Explícitas)* promotes equal access to healthcare for a specific list of health problems, which is being progressively expanded in subsequent years. Although the Chilean health reforms were intended to encourage a more preventive approach to healthcare, as in other nations NGOs have never been viewed as potential resources in the health arena by reformers.

Health sector reform has been far less extensive in Uruguay than in Chile, although some subsidies to the private sector have been provided to help offset the rapidly rising cost of public healthcare. Approximately 45% of the population receives healthcare through the public sector. However, even as the cost of supporting the public sector has increased, the quality of services has deteriorated and is generally viewed as markedly inferior to that in the private sector. The private sector consists primarily of non-profit institutions known as *Instituciones de Asistencia Médica Colectiva* (IAMCs), more commonly referred as *mutualistas*, that cover more than half of all Uruguayans, including the middle class and those with formal employment. These organisations, which originated as small groups of professional cooperatives and migrants associations, are financed by contributions from the social security system to which employers and workers contribute. A growing number of middle-class Uruguayans are purchasing private supplemental health insurance plans to supplement IAMC coverage (World Bank, 2005).

The expansion of the IAMC system in the 1970s and 1980s and the massive enrolment of new subscribers have resulted in serious structural and financial problems that have made substantial public subsidies necessary. The economic crisis of the late 1990s and the rise in the number of unemployed people who no longer pay into the social security system have had a major impact on the revenues of the *mutualistas*, which have lost a large number of subscribers in recent years (Ramos, 2004). As a consequence, many IAMCs have failed and the system is facing the most serious fiscal crisis in its history. Although some modest reforms have been introduced, the rejection of more basic restructuring by the state has resulted in growing inequity in access to healthcare and an increasing gap in quality between public and public services. In the absence of large-scale healthcare system reform, the preservation of benefits for the middle class has come at the cost of deteriorating care for the poor. One of the greatest challenges for the recently elected socialist government is the development of an equitable and universal national health insurance plan. Once again, though, there has been little discussion at the national level of the potential role of NGOs in health maintenance or healthcare.

Identification and selection of NGOs for field interviews

Our fieldwork on Chilean and Uruguayan NGOs – in the cities of Santiago in Chile and Montevideo in Uruguay – consisted of interviews with key informants, including public officials, academics and NGO administrators, as well as observation of staff and meetings. The initial challenge was to define and identify the universe of health-related NGOs. We began by developing an extensive list of organisations that engaged in some preventive, supportive or other health-related service or activity, either as advocates or as service providers. This master list was developed from local directories, lists of public programmes, NGO registries and other secondary sources that provided information for use by clients and organisations seeking information about resources available in the community. Although these sources did not provide in-depth information concerning the organisations, they provided a reliable source for identifying organisations, finding contact information and identifying the organisations' major activities.

In both cities there were many social programmes run by public agencies, municipalities or both that included NGOs as contractual partners for the delivery of public services. The directors and officials of these programmes provided invaluable information for the identification of and access to NGOs involved in health services broadly defined. Additionally, active national associations of NGOs (two in Chile and one in Uruguay) provided registries with basic information concerning their member organisations. In some instances these national-level associations had conducted profile studies and in-depth analysis of the changing characteristics of their affiliated organisations (Morgan, 2001). These studies were very useful secondary sources of information. Once organisations were identified and an initial contact made with one agency, a snowball sampling procedure was used to contact other organisations. This procedure fairly quickly provided information concerning the universe of local organisations in each city.

Allies of the state in service delivery

The role of NGOs in relation to the state can be usefully characterised according to the degree of correspondence between the objectives of NGOs in a particular sector and the needs and policies of the state in relation to non-state actors. An NGO, or the movement as a whole, may assume the role of *ally* of the state in dealing with particular problem areas, or it can position itself as an *adversary* of the state, depending on state policies and the sources and nature of the social problems to be addressed. This dichotomy of ally versus adversary of course misrepresents a complex reality since, although NGOs often originated in an opposition to specific state policies or to address state shortcomings, democratisation and the decentralisation of state functions have profoundly changed the political arena in which these organisations operate in Chile and Uruguay, as well as many other nations in Latin America. Nonetheless, the distinction provides a rhetorical and theoretical starting point.

In the current political environment the characterisation of the degree of state/NGO cooperation offers some utility in explaining the political meaning of NGO initiatives as well as their programme effectiveness. One might usefully characterise NGOs as *allies* of the state when they cooperate with state agencies in achieving public goals through the provision of specific services. In contrast, NGOs assume the role of *adversaries* when their primary goal is to hold the state accountable in terms of carrying out universal mandates, including those of assuring the political rights and material welfare of disadvantaged groups. The adversarial role involves promoting changes in specific state policies and assuring transparency in the ways in which policies are developed and implemented.

As is the case with most complex social movements and organisations, our research reveals that these two positions are not mutually exclusive and that, in fact, they are often combined within the same organisational setting, sometimes at different points in the organisation's life cycle, and sometimes in different organisational subunits. Often a particular organisation may be uncertain about whether to position itself as an ally or adversary of the state, or may change its position within a relatively short period of time in response to changing circumstances. A staff meeting of *Casa Lunas*, an NGO providing services for teenage mothers in the outskirts of Montevideo, serves as an example of what can become an ongoing conflict between these two identities. The NGO's primary objective is to provide support to teenage mothers and reduce teenage pregnancy rates. At one meeting the discussion revolved around the issue of whether or not to submit a proposal for a new project to the Uruguayan government to be funded with a loan from the International Development Bank (IDB). The discussion took on a profoundly ideological character as the participants debated the political meaning and consequences of their decision and what it meant to 'work with' the state and 'cooperate with' the IDB on a project that had clear political implications. As noted by Acuña (2003), NGOs often take contradictory positions with respect to multilateral development banks, just as they often do with respect to states. The NGO world tends to be ideologically separated to varying degrees into those who mistrust states and multilateral agencies, which are often seen as state allies, and those who see cooperation as a means of influencing their actions. In fact, we observed that conflicts between the roles of ally and adversary operate both between and within organisations. At any one moment, some programmes or departments might be working in conjunction with the state, while others might be challenging state policy and advocating for the rights of a specific group.

Generally, the organisations that assume the role of adversaries of the state tend to focus their efforts on the process of agenda setting and policy formulation in an attempt to influence the ways in which issues are framed for the purpose of policy development. These organisations engage in political activities that are aimed at the introduction of new models for the enforcement of formal rights. Organisations that assume the role of adversaries, then, complement the efforts of organisations that function as allies of the state. As part of their advocacy activities, adversary organisations contribute to promoting the rights of minority ethnic and marginalised groups through expanding awareness of their plight, and by mobilising efforts on their behalf to hold the state accountable.

The increasingly important role of NGOs as allies of the state holds great potential for effective action in terms of:

- direct service delivery;
- capacity building at local and municipal levels;
- demonstration projects.

In the realm of training and capacity building, the data reveal great potential for NGOs in the role of assisting the state in particular situations. We encountered situations in which non-governmental personnel supported and trained public officials to provide services. The example of the government health clinic *Santa Rita* in Casavalle, one of the poorest urban neighbourhoods in Montevideo, reveals the potential for problem solving that is possible when this type of public–private partnership is successful. The clinic and its staff had been the subjects of aggressive actions and threats by local residents and the director was seriously considering closing the clinic or moving it out of the area. Before doing so the director decided to request the assistance of a local NGO, *El Abrojo*, with knowledge of the community and experience in serving the needs of marginal groups. This NGO was able to provide the health team with new insights into the episodes of violence against the centre and enable the team to reopen the service.

A growing NGO presence in health

Our research revealed a significant presence of NGOs in several domains including:

- HIV/AIDS;
- sexual and reproductive health;
- drug abuse prevention/rehabilitation;
- mental health services;
- elder care;
- child and maternal healthcare.

We also identified NGOs that are dealing with specific populations and organisations that exist in an ambiguous location between the state and civil society. These include:

- organisations that deal with the needs of indigenous populations and advocate for cultural specificities in health (for example Mapuche healthcare needs in Chile);
- organisations that monitor public services in order to assure that the quality of the care they provide is adequate;
- primary healthcare clinics that have been fully transferred to NGO administration although they remain within the public system.

Even this brief and almost certainly incomplete inventory reveals a wealth of health-related activity carried out by NGOs, often as only a part of their overall agendas.

The first question that comes to mind is: what do these areas have in common that makes them the focus of NGO intervention? Additionally, it seems important to identify those aspects of NGO structure and function that make them particularly well suited for these specific missions. Unfortunately, the literature offers little theoretical or empirical guidance, and it was clear that beyond the classification of types of NGO activities, a more grounded theoretical elaboration of the relationship between the structure and function of NGOs, as well as their relationship to the state, is called for. In what follows we present a grounded theoretical model of NGO activity in the health sector that focuses on state shortcomings and NGO strengths to begin to understand the growth of this organisational form in certain problem areas. Ultimately, our objective is to develop a theoretical model that might lead to broader discussions concerning the effectiveness of NGOs of various forms in dealing with specific problem domains.

We begin with one obvious explanation for the concentration of NGO efforts in the problem areas we identified. This has to do with the limitations and constraints that states encounter in providing fairly routine services to large numbers of individuals, as well as the fact that the non-governmental sector demonstrates certain advantages in the delivery of such routine services to specific populations. Non-governmental organisations rarely provide expensive or highly technical surgical or other tertiary care. Rather, they focus their efforts on preventive, supportive and other low-cost routine interventions that complement the state health delivery system. Table 7.1, which is based on our preliminary observations, presents a list of state and NGO characteristics that helps explain the social locations in which NGOs emerge and persist. In general, we found a higher concentration of NGOs in situations where the state's role is characterised by one or more of the conditions listed in the left-hand column of Table 7.1. Concurrently, we found that the characteristics listed in the right-hand column of Table 7.1 related to the organisation being associated with a high probability of NGO entry and persistence.

As Table 7.1 suggests, certain problem areas emerge in which at a particular historical moment and in a particular culture the state lacks adequate knowledge of the problem area or of the population at risk, as in the case of minority ethnic communities, or it has insufficient legitimacy to intervene, as in the case of the

Table 7.1: State and non-governmental organisational characteristics that determine the domains within which NGOs function effectively

State shortcomings or incapacities	NGO capacities
The state is unable to formulate new approaches or intervention strategies for specific groups (eg culturally appropriate care)	The NGO possesses knowledge of and can work with special populations
The state lacks sufficient legitimate authority to introduce new approaches or is unable to adapt quickly	The NGO can adopt new and effective but potentially controversial approaches
The state lacks trained personnel or the human resources with which to address a problem area	The NGO is sufficiently professionalised and has adequate expertise in a problem area
The state needs to extend coverage to a large number of people and lacks the economic resources	The NGO has a proven adequate resource-generating capacity

distribution of syringes for HIV prevention. In these situations the state often also lacks the expertise or the personnel to address the problem. In many of these same cases the needs are technically simple but extensive and affect a large number of people. In many cases the state simply lacks the resources to address the full range of the problem. As Table 7.1 indicates, when the NGO has the expertise, staffing and resources, it can address at least a part of the problem and complement state efforts. Together, such organisations constitute a major social resource for addressing problem areas that might otherwise be ignored. In what follows we employ Table 7.1 as a means of understanding the origin, role and relationship to the state of some of the NGOs we studied.

We must, of course, avoid simplifications and stereotypes. The extreme characterisation of a bureaucratic, rigid and slow state, in contrast to a professional, flexible and efficient NGO sector, is merely heuristic. What we encounter in fact are traits and characteristics that appertain to certain problem domains and that are possessed by organisations to varying degrees. These traits and characteristics of problem domains and organisations serve as plausible explanations for the presence or absence of NGO forms in specific subfields of healthcare.

One extreme manifestation of the changing roles of the state and private organisations was revealed in Santiago by a few cases in which health clinics that were part of the public network of care providers had been administratively transferred to NGOs. Although the phenomenon was limited, we found cases of NGOs assuming direct responsibility for a small number of clinics that remained part of the public network. These NGOs are paid based on the same criteria that municipal or health ministries apply in the allocation of resources to their own providers. However, like most third sector organisations, these services also take advantage of their institutional capacity to collect funds from alternative sources.

Primary health clinics, like the one run by the NGO *Cristo Vive* in the low-income *comuna* of Ricoleta, Chile, provide ambulatory services based on a family approach to community needs. These clinics offer medical services for children and adults, prenatal care, contraceptive education, dental care, mental health services and other specialised services. Although we encountered only a handful of such cases, the fact that the experiment has begun suggests that governments may be more open to increasing the responsibility of NGOs in the direct provision of primary health services as they face more serious fiscal constraints.

A model of NGO activity in the health sector

Perhaps we can best summarise the question of 'where does one find healthcare NGOs?' with the simple reply, 'where the state needs them'. If the growing NGO presence and activity during the 1970s and 1980s was largely motivated by opposition to state repression and the neglect of social needs, it has evolved into something quite different in the health arena. In their daily operation NGOs are increasingly complementary to the state. Of course, healthcare NGOs have not emerged in a vacuum and their development and mission have been constrained by the actions of the state and the particular needs of the communities they serve, both of which limit their abilities for autonomous action. From our observations it seems clear that NGOs function in what we might label the periphery of the health service delivery sector. They play a clear subsidiary role relative to the state. In Chile, as in Uruguay, a traditionally strong public health system assures that NGOs continue to play a secondary role in health services. This fact is both inevitable and probably desirable given the requirement that the paternalistic state provide basic healthcare to its citizens.

In both Chile and Uruguay, medical care, especially for low-income citizens, is provided by public health networks and relatively few NGOs are involved in providing acute healthcare. Rather, they focus on ancillary, auxiliary or post-acute support services that are an indispensable part of any comprehensive healthcare system, but that are not provided, or are not provided in adequate amounts, within the formal healthcare system. In general terms our observations lead us to the observation that NGO activities tend to focus on issues related to 'community health' broadly defined, and for the most part these organisations engage in an array of actions related to health promotion, illness prevention and health education. Such services can be provided at relatively low cost, but provide great hope for improving community and population health levels.

Our interviews clearly showed that the health sector is dynamic and that the role of NGOs in providing services is evolving in response to changes in population health profiles and healthcare needs, changes in the role of the state in relation to the financing and provision of healthcare and changes in the healthcare marketplace itself. Non-profit charitable organisations, which have always ministered to the poor and the sick, find themselves assuming new and more extensive roles as health problems that might have been ignored in the past become socially and politically salient. New diseases or old social problems that have become more salient including HIV/AIDS, drug abuse and the chronic conditions that inevitably accompany the ageing of populations create the need for extensive educational and support services. The decentralisation of administrative control and demands for the social rights of vulnerable populations give rise to new healthcare demands that states are often ill-equipped to address. Increasingly, the NGO is a significant player in this new arena largely, as we have seen, because it possesses accumulated expertise in providing basic services to hard-to-reach populations and the most desperately needy.

Clearly, NGOs cannot replace the state in providing basic healthcare and critics of the increasing presence of NGOs in healthcare might fault them for letting states off the hook by giving the impression that health problems that only the state can deal with are being addressed. As we have emphasised, the NGO mission in the developing world, as it is in the developed world, remains largely supportive and confined to the periphery of healthcare delivery where these organisations provide ancillary services. Their presence in no way absolves the state of the responsibility for providing basic healthcare to its citizens.

Perhaps, though, the unclear distinction between state-sponsored and non-governmental organisations and the similar fuzzy distinction between for-profit and non-profit enterprises brings us to the issue of the analytic and practical utility of the NGO classification. From our observations the category is so heterogeneous and the ties to both states and the market so common and pervasive that only the most core 'northern' NGOs lend themselves to easy classification. The category might even be usefully conceived of as a residual category that includes any organisation or activity that cannot be unambiguously classified as either a state-sponsored and administered enterprise or a market-oriented activity. In the healthcare arena there are many such organisations with fuzzy boundaries and changing and fluid missions. Increasing variety of new institutional arrangements created at the frontiers of the state and the market, such as state-dependent private NGOs or private corporations of public interests created by municipal governments, challenge the authenticity or conceptual autonomy of a third sector.

We suspect that typologies of such organisations, or even clear distinctions among governmental, for-profit and non-governmental/non-profit organisations, may prove to be of less utility that one might initially hope. Unlike botany, the starting point for understanding the NGO domain may not be classification. The forms and activities of the organisations in this domain are too varied and changing to lend themselves to categorisation. After all, if what we need is conceptual equipment that enables us to understand the expansion of these new institutional expressions, their effectiveness and their contribution to longlasting social and political change, the creation of a separate third sector that operates outside the margins of the state and the market may impoverish more than enhance our understanding.

Our foray into the domain of NGO activity in healthcare tells us much about the potential role of the organisations of civil society for addressing increasingly complex social problems generally. Education, human rights, gender equality, sustainable development and much more represent areas in which the state's role is central, but limited in terms of the ability of any government to provide the full range of needed services to all citizens. In these areas NGOs continue to combine their roles as adversaries who demand government accountability and allies who join in the effort to reach collective ends. Even relatively modest reductions in inequality require massive transfers of wealth to the poor and the NGO might represent one mechanism for doing so in relatively peaceful and politically acceptable ways. Whatever their long-term form, in the area of healthcare delivery and support, NGOs are clearly a permanent reality. They will operate in increasingly complex health delivery environments that, as in Chile today, consist of one or more public sectors and a private sector with government-sponsored and recognised service providers some of which are formally non-profit. As a consequence, even today NGOs are becoming highly professionalised and savvy at the game of fundraising in complex political and economic environments in which they face multiple competitors.

New challenges for state–NGO linkages

Although the NGO presence in healthcare is becoming more widespread, potential problems with an excessive reliance on the non-governmental sector must be acknowledged. When NGOs find themselves in the position of appearing to compensate for state failures in providing basic social services they can divert attention from the need to increase state capacity. Since NGOs are motivated by the same survival logic as other organisations, they can become preoccupied with their own organisational survival and lose sight of the need to transfer accumulated knowledge and share novel models of intervention both with the state and other organisations. During the years of dictatorship in Chile and Uruguay the NGO community largely rejected the idea of collaboration with the state. Since the return of democratic regimes, such collaboration has become both possible and desirable. Through public–private initiatives, NGOs might help avoid regressive effects that could worsen the situation of those who need services (Castells, 1998). As we have seen, although they cannot replace the state in providing the full range of healthcare to populations, NGOs often enjoy more flexibility and political autonomy than state agencies, and they are often in a better position to experiment with innovative interventions.

In the end we are left with two basic questions that form the basis for an ongoing discourse on the role of civil society in healthcare in Latin America. Perhaps the most obvious question relates to how civil society in general can intervene in the provision of social services generally without lessening state capacity or responsibility for providing basic human services. On the other hand, the opposite concern leads us to ask how the state can function in ways that take advantage of NGO capacities and that do not weaken civil society organisations. The health sector offers unique opportunities for investigating the possible answers to these questions. Although they are at different points in the process, both Chile and Uruguay have introduced basic healthcare reforms with the common objective of increasing equity in access to quality healthcare. A fundamental motivation for these reforms is the fact that public health systems are simply not able to respond to increasing demand. Re-establishing the state's capacity to provide basic services was a fundamental goal of the Lagos administration in Chile and represents one of the major challenges faced by President Tabare Vazquez in Uruguay. Unfortunately, in neither country has the more extensive and coordinated use of civil society organisations been seriously considered as a key aspect of formal healthcare sector reform. Our continuing research mandate is to better understand why greater use of this potential resource has not been made and how it might be.

References

Acuña, C. (2003) 'La participación comunitaria en el Programa Materno Infantil y Nutrición (PROMIN) de la Argentina: Una asignatura en gran medida pendiente', in I. González Bombal and R.Villar (eds) *Organizaciones de la Sociedad Civil e Incidencia en Políticas Públicas*, Buenos Aires: Libros del Zorzal.

Benett, J. and Gibbs, S. (1996) *NGO funding strategies: an introduction for southern and eastern NGOs*, Oxford: INTRAC.

Boli, J. and Thomas, G.M. (1999) *World polity formation since 1875: World culture and international non-governmental organizations*, Stanford, CA: Stanford University Press.

Castells, M. (1998) *The information age: Economy, society and culture, Vol III: End of millennium,* Malden, MA, and Oxford: Blackwell Publishers.

Clark, J. (1991) *Democratizing development: The role of voluntary organizations,* West Hartford, CT: Kumarian Press.

Cruz-Saco, M.A. and Mesa-Lago, C. (eds) (1999) *Do options exist? The reform of pension and healthcare systems in Latin America,* Pittsburgh, PA: University of Pittsburgh Press.

De la Maza, G. and Ochsenius, C. (2001) 'Acción Internacional de las Redes No Gubernamentales Latinoamericanas: Reflejo o superposición a las realidades nacionales?', Unpublished manuscript.

DeJong, J. (2003) *Making an impact in HIV and AIDS: NGO experiences of scaling up,* London: ITDG Publishing.

Edwards, M. and Hulme, D. (eds) (1996) *Beyond the magic bullet: NGO performance and accountability in the post-Cold War world,* West Hartford, CT: Kumarian.

Fowler, A. (1988) 'Non-governmental organizations in Africa: achieving comparative advantage in relief and micro-development', Discussion Paper No 249, Brighton: Institute of Development Studies.

Fox, J. and Aranda, J. (1996) *Decentralization and rural development in Mexico: Community participation in Oaxaca's Municipal Funds Program,* San Diego, CA: Center for US–Mexican Studies, University of California.

Gais, T., Burke, C. and Corso, R. (2003) *A divided community: The effects of state fiscal crises on non-profits providing health and social assistance,* Albany, NY: Rockefeller Institute.

Mesa-Lago, C. and Amparo Cruz-Saco, M. (eds) (1999) *The reform of pension and health care systems in Latin America,* Pittsburgh, PA: Pittsburgh University Press.

Meyer, J. and Hannan, M. (eds) (1979) *National development and the world system,* Chicago, IL: University of Chicago Press.

Miranda, E. (1994) *La Salud en Chile: Evolución y perspectivas,* Santiago: Centro de Estudios Públicos.

Morgan, M. de la L. (2001) *Situación de las ONGs Chilenas al inicio del Siglo XXI,* Santiago: Acción, Asociación Chilena de ONGs.

Pearce, J. (1993) 'NGOs and social change: agents or facilitators?', *Development in Practice* 3(3): 222-7.

Prud'homme, R. (1995) 'The dangers of decentralization', *The World Bank Research Observer* 10(2): 201-20.

Ramos, A. (2004) 'Análisis del Mercado de Salud Privado del Uruguay', Montevideo, Unpublished manuscript.

Renshaw, L.R. (1994) 'Strengthening civil society', *Development* 4: 46-9.

Salamon, L. and Anheier, H. (1994) *The emerging sector: An overview*, Baltimore, MD: Johns Hopkins University.

Salamon, L. and Anheier, H. (1998) 'Social origins of civil society: explaining the nonprofit sector cross-nationally', *Voluntas: International Journal of Voluntary and Nonprofit Organizations* 9(3): 213-48.

Salamon, L. and Anheier, H. (1999) *The emerging sector revisited: A summary*, Baltimore, MD: Johns Hopkins University.

Thomas, G., Meyer, J., Ramirez, F. and Boli, J. (eds) (1987) *Institutional structure: Constituting state, society, and individual*, Newbury Park, CA: Sage Publications.

Twombly, E.C. (2001) *Welfare reform's impact on the failure rate of nonprofit human service providers*, Washington, DC: The Urban Institute.

UNAIDS (United Nations Joint Programme on HIV/AIDS) (2002) *Report on the global HIV/AIDS epidemic*, Geneva: UNAIDS.

Willis, E., Garman, C. and Haggard, S. (1999) 'The politics of decentralization in Latin America', *Latin American Research Review* 34(1): 7-50.

World Bank (2005) *Private and public initiatives: Working together in health and education*, Washington, DC: World Bank.

Pathway 3
Psychosocial factors in individual health

Health inequalities and the role of psychosocial work factors: the Whitehall II Study

Eric Brunner

Introduction

Despite the improvements in average income, life continues to be a struggle for many people. Although Marx has not proved to be the inspiration for vibrant social development, his concept of alienation resonates today. As social commentator Terry Eagleton has observed, alienation is embedded in the post-soviet, market-driven world (Eagleton, 2003). Culture and values are now important commodities, not so much in the marketplace, as the very fabric of the marketplace. Without wealth and money it is impossible to participate in the range of activities that the mass media constantly reflect to us: prestige is all too present in our consciousness.

The experience of 'stress' is in some ways a clear demand for these social values to be overturned. Health has improved – but social inequalities in health are growing: on the one hand, shell suits, trainers and unemployment in Workington in Cumbria (North West England) where the steel mill is about to close after 134 years of production, on the other, Armani, Mercedes and five-figure bonuses in the wealthy suburb of Richmond, London. Along with these extremes of wealth, there is a four-year life expectancy gap and a 16-year difference in *healthy* life expectancy (Bajekal, 2005). So who is most likely to suffer from stress? In my example, is it the former or the latter? Of course, it is the former, echoing the concept of alienation: a feeling, as New Labour politicians used to put it, that 'I am not a stakeholder'.

Psychoanalysts recognise that an inability to suppress anxiety and antagonism can destabilise close relationships. Such dynamics can be considered to contribute to racism, community violence and other types of dysfunctional behaviour, which often emerge in deprived rather than wealthy communities. These are the manifestations of the time-honoured struggle for resources, and their psychological consequences.

For the large proportion of the population who do not lack the basic, material requirements for living, a different set of problems and preoccupations exist.

Relative deprivation and health

Most of us have never known absolute poverty, yet constant well-being remains elusive. Richard Layard (2005) and Daniel Kahneman (Kahneman et al, 2003) have studied the link between economic trends and the emotional state of the nations. In the US, average GDP per head more than doubled in the past 50 years, but happiness (% 'very happy') has remained quite constant at about 35%, with no decline in the proportion 'not too happy' (12%, according to the General Social Survey).

In the US, recent surveys show that roughly 14% of people aged 35 have experienced a clinical depression. At any one time about 2% of the population suffers from depression, and many experience it recurrently. In comparison, only 2% of Americans had experienced depression by age 35 in the 1950s. In the UK, depression qualifies as a major public health problem, with an annual incidence of 8–12%. Reduction in quality of life is comparable to that seen in major chronic physical diseases, and the economic consequences of depression are profound: US$14 billion (£8 billion) each year in the UK and US$83 billion (£50 billion) in the US (Gilbody et al, 2006).

On the basis of these population trends, the quest for happiness and pleasure through market-driven economic growth seems to be a flawed enterprise. Put another way, the utilitarian project that seeks to maximise the sum of happiness in society is most unlikely to succeed because it fails to take account of the nature of social hierarchy. There is a human preference for a balance between order and liberty, which leads to a number of conditions:

- first, there is some form of social hierarchy, which in its starkest manifestation places legitimate violence and use of force entirely in the hands of the state;
- second, social conflict is institutionalised and can lead to political and legislative change in a healthy society;
- third, when social reciprocity, the balance between rights and responsibilities, is considered to have been lost by even a significant minority, social disruption and unhappiness are likely to follow.

Political conceptions of a healthy society

Richard Tawney (1880–1962; LSE Professor of Economic History 1931–49) was a British democratic socialist who recognised some of the limitations of economic self-interest:

> No individual can create by his isolated actions a healthy environment, or establish an education system ... or organise an industry ... to diminish economic insecurity.... Yet these are the conditions which make the difference between happiness and misery ... life and death....

In so far as they exist they are a source of social income received not in the form of money, but of increased well-being.

The concept of the social contract was developed by another political philosopher, John Rawls (1921–2002; Harvard University, 1962–94). He addressed the question of distribution in *A theory of justice* (Rawls, 1971) by elaborating a liberal position that linked social justice with a degree of economic fairness. These two principles can be summarised as follows: (1) equality in the assignment of basic rights and duties, and (2) social and economic inequalities, for example wealth and authority are just only if they result in compensating benefits for everyone, and in particular for the least advantaged.

These thoughts lead us to consider the nature of work, the environment in which we spend much of our adult life while outside the home, and from which we gain much of our social standing and recognition, and our wage, provided we are not unemployed. Conditions of work are a reflection of wider social values, shaped by culture and legislation. In small, medium and large organisations there is generally a hierarchy of experience and pay that constitutes a key social role and focus of modern life.

Autonomy, reciprocity and fairness in the work hierarchy

Social epidemiology seeks to quantify the nature of work hierarchies and to investigate the relation to health. There are two dominant models of psychosocial work characteristics. Both are based on self-completion questionnaires with around 20 questions each. First, the Karasek-Theorell model dates to the 1970s and has two main dimensions: demands and control (Theorell and Floderus-Myrhed, 1977; Karasek and Theorell, 1990). This 'job strain' model is intuitively meaningful. High strain is experienced by those reporting high work demands and a low level of control (decision latitude/autonomy). Production line and call-centre workers and supermarket checkout operators fit this type of work experience. At the other extreme, high control and low demands, classed as low strain, may be the luck of the old-fashioned ivory tower academic. High control plus high demands is the lot of senior professionals, for example doctors and lawyers, and is known as 'active work'. Passive work is characterised by low demands and low control. Shop assistants and receptionists may have this work experience. A third dimension, social support at work, is sometimes added to the job strain model. This measures the feeling of isolation in the workplace, with questions on support from colleagues and supervisors, which together with job strain generates the concept of 'iso-strain'.

Second, Siegrist's job stress model, now some 15 years old, has a different focus. The notion of social reciprocity in interpersonal behaviour is important in the effort–reward imbalance model (Siegrist, 1996). Social reciprocity is characterised by mutual cooperative investments based on the expectation that efforts are equalised by material and psychological rewards to each party, employee and employer. Failed reciprocity resulting from a violation of this norm elicits negative emotions because it threatens this fundamental principle. Conversely, positive emotions evoked by appropriate social rewards promote well-being. Individuals and groups may find themselves with little latitude for selecting their experience in the labour market. Work contracts may be poorly defined or employees have little choice of alternative work due to low level of skill, lack of mobility or a precarious labour market. Employees may accept effort–reward imbalance temporarily for strategic reasons, for instance to improve future work prospects by anticipatory investments. Experience of high-cost–low-gain work is common among individuals who exhibit a cognitive and motivational pattern of coping with demands characterised by excessive work-related involvement ('overcommitment').

One way to think about the difference between these two work stress models is to see self-reports of control and demands as an evaluation of how the organisation treats the worker. On the other hand, effort and reward reflect the way a worker feels about the employer.

The social contract played out in the workplace reflects important dimensions of the hierarchy that underlies relative deprivation. Material hardship is present for individuals and their families in low-paid work. For others, growing wage differentials reinforce the sense of position in the occupational hierarchy above the subsistence level. In addition, the psychosocial dimensions of work, including demand, control, effort and psychological reward, further define social position and create the context for socioeconomic inequality to get under the skin. There is a strong parallel between the classification of occupation in terms of power and autonomy, and the Marxist concept of class. The approach is the basis for the Erikson–Goldthorpe class schema, which provides the framework for the new British socioeconomic classification (Erikson and Goldthorpe, 1992). Position in the occupational hierarchy may influence health by several pathways involving material resources, self-esteem, social (dis)approval and behavioural patterns.

Hierarchy, distress and depression

One expectation that flows from our perspective of a parallel between social hierarchy and work hierarchy is that there will be an occupational gradient in distress, as there is in the general population, and that the psychosocial characteristics of work will have a major explanatory role. This is the case in the British civil service. Using a four-item depression subscale from the 30-item General Health Questionnaire, the prevalence of depressive symptoms increased from 9% in the highest administrator grade to 22% in the clerical grade among men in the Whitehall II Study at phase 5 (1997–99). Among women the prevalence was 11% among administrators and 17% in the clerical grade (Stansfeld et al, 2003).

In men, work characteristics provided the best statistical explanation of the occupational gradient in depressive symptoms. When job control, job demands, work social support and effort–reward imbalance were controlled for, the occupational gradient was reduced by two thirds (66% reduction of slope coefficient) compared to material problems (25%), social support outside work (21%) and health behaviours (15%). In women, material problems and work characteristics accounted for similar proportions of the gradient (47% and 43% respectively). The gender difference, with material problems more important in women and work characteristics more important in men, probably reflects the unequal location of women in lower grades and men in higher grades, leading to income inequity, and potentially the higher priority given to the work role by men.

Common mental disorder is inversely related to occupational status, and adverse psychosocial work environment accounts for a part of this gradient. Considering the political philosophers' argument that well-being (and other dimensions of population health) is dependent not only on economic growth but also on social justice, the evidence from Whitehall II Study is highly supportive. The key elements of social and relational justice are embedded within the job stress questionnaire items (Table 8.1). These elements are autonomy, fairness and respect. Their importance extends into all social roles, and therefore we can see that investigations of psychosocial effects on health within occupational hierarchies are relevant to non-work contexts.

Physical disease: the disputed ground

It is not remarkable to find that organisational injustice at work influences psychological health. The disputed territory relates to the role of work psychosocial factors ('stress') in producing physical disease. Behavioural explanations dominate in conventional medical thinking, while social scientists, social epidemiologists

Table 8.1: Organisational justice and fairness items within the Karasek-Theorell job strain and Siegrist effort–reward imbalance questionnaires

Karasek-Theorell job strain questionnaire items
Do you ever get praised for your work?
Do you ever get criticised unfairly?
Do you get sufficient information from line management (your superiors)?
Do you get consistent information from line management (your superiors)?
How often do you get help and support from your immediate superior?
How often is your immediate superior willing to listen to your problems?
Siegrist effort–reward imbalance questionnaire items
I receive the respect I deserve from my superiors.
I am treated unfairly at work.
Considering all my efforts and achievements, I receive the respect and prestige I deserve at work.

included, are divided between those favouring neo-materialist explanations and those interested in the processes that translate socioeconomic inequality into biological risk. The Whitehall II Study has been tackling *social-biological translation* since it began. The physical health outcomes under study are heart attack and other manifestations of coronary heart disease (CHD), diabetes and their respective precursors.

The senior sociologist Mildred Blaxter observed that researchers in the field of health inequalities find studying biology an awkward approach to explanation. While it is usual to measure social phenomena on the one hand and health on the other, the intervening processes tend to be avoided. There are at least two reasons for this avoidance: the danger of distraction from the social roots of health inequalities, and an antipathy to the 'biomedical model'. Sociology has tended to distance itself from the body. But we should not abstain, but recognise that social inequalities must generate biological inequalities.

The value of studying the biology of health inequalities is that inequalities translate into disease via differences in fashions and aspirations and material resources, leading literally to the embodiment of social class. The very different experiences of health and illness across social strata mean we can be certain that a barrister's body is not the same as a hairdresser's or a bus driver's body. This proves to be true even within the ranks of the civil service.

The Whitehall studies

The first Whitehall study showed that inequalities in health were not limited to the health consequences of poverty. Important as that issue remains, the Whitehall question was why there should be a social gradient in disease in people above the poverty threshold. Conventional risk factors (smoking, blood cholesterol, blood pressure) were an imperfect explanation of the mortality risk differential between the clerical and administrative grades, and much of it remained unexplained (Marmot et al, 1984). Mortality gradients in the study were in the same direction as national social class mortality data, but larger.

The Whitehall II Study, a longitudinal study of British civil servants, was started in 1985 with the intention of examining reasons for the social gradient in health and disease in men and extending the research to include women (Marmot and Brunner, 2005). The theoretical perspective places wider determinants of health within the causal framework, adding material and psychosocial context to the narrower biomedical model that tended to underpin cohort studies of cardiovascular disease until the 1980s.

The target population for the Whitehall II Study was all civil servants aged 35 to 55 years working in the London offices of 20 Whitehall departments in 1985-88. The achieved sample size was 10,308 people: 3,413 women and 6,895 men. The participants, who were from clerical and office support grades, middle-ranking executive grades and senior administrative grades, differed widely in salary. Annual salary ranges for these three groups of workers were £7,387–£11,917,

£8,517–£25,554 and £25,330–£87,620 respectively on 1 August 1992. Some have remained in the civil service. Many have retired, others have taken employment elsewhere and some are now unemployed. The participants have been followed up nine times to date. The whole cohort is invited to the research clinic at five-year intervals, and a postal questionnaire is sent to participants between clinic phases.

Our research model focuses on two types of pathway. One connects psychosocial stress factors directly to biological changes that increase risk of illness. The second places behaviour patterns of smoking, diet, exercise and alcohol consumption on the pathway between stress factors and disease. Figure 8.1 illustrates the model in schematic terms. Until we have shown biological mechanisms by which psychosocial factors act to cause heart disease and other diseases, we cannot claim to have demonstrated causation. The analytic strategy is to examine the extent to which the pathways we identify account statistically for the social gradient in incident disease.

Social position predicts CHD, with biological and behavioural mediators

Socioeconomic position (measured by employment grade) is inversely associated with validated fatal and non-fatal CHD events from baseline (1985–88) to the end of 1999. The hazard ratio between bottom and top ends of the employment grade spectrum is 2.1 in men and 2.0 in women. Biological variables related to the metabolic syndrome (obesity, high blood pressure, glucose intolerance, low high-density lipoprotein (HDL) cholesterol, high triglyceride level) and plasma fibrinogen account for about half of the social gradient in CHD. In our low smoking prevalence cohort, pack-years exposure based on three study phases of data account for 22% of the social gradient in fatal CHD/non-fatal myocardial

Figure 8.1: Schematic model: direct and indirect pathways linking psychosocial factors to illness

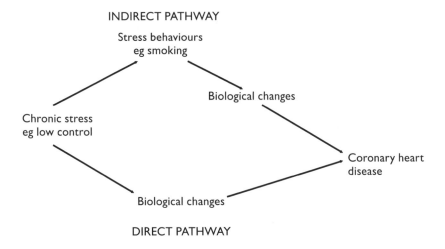

infarction (MI). Dietary patterns identified by cluster analysis (Martikainen et al, 2003) and physical activity (Rennie et al, 2003), each contribute to the social gradient in metabolic syndrome. Together with behavioural factors (smoking, physical activity and alcohol) and height, we could account for two thirds of the gradient.

Social position, diabetes and health-related functioning

There are significant age-adjusted social gradients in incident diabetes (Figure 8.2) and physical functioning, assessed with the SF-36 (a short-form health survey with 36 questions) (Figure 8.3). These contrasting measures of health both show strong stepwise inequalities. An important observation is that when those with incident disease are removed from the analysis, the inverse social gradient in physical functioning remains. This implies that it is not entirely the result of disease. Physical functioning declines with age, but the effect is stronger in lower-grade men. This finding suggests that the passage of time does not have the same consequences for everyone, and that the influence of social environment as well as biology, is at work.

Direct stress effects

Well-known candidate biological mechanisms exist that may link psychosocial factors to cardiovascular disease (CVD) risk. The common feature is that the mechanisms involve a homeostatic system such as that controlling blood sugar level. Repeated challenges may produce permanent or reversible adverse changes in the

Figure 8.2: Incidence of Type 2 diabetes by employment grade

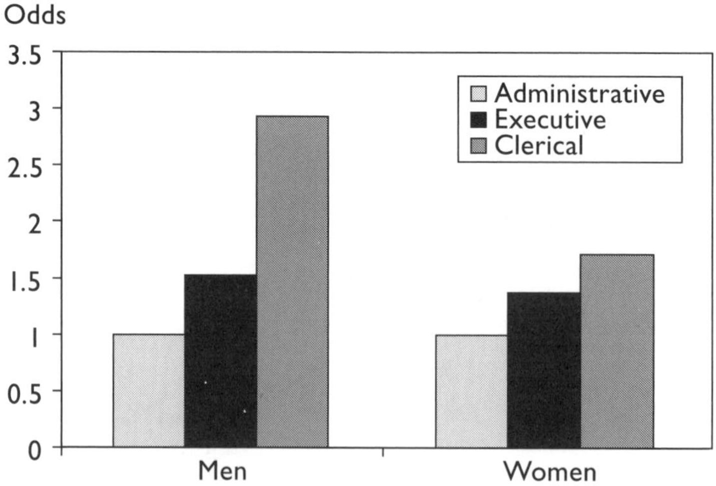

Note: Odds ratio adjusted for age and length of follow-up

Source: Kumari et al (2004)

Figure 8.3: SF-36 physical function by employment grade (Whitehall II Study)

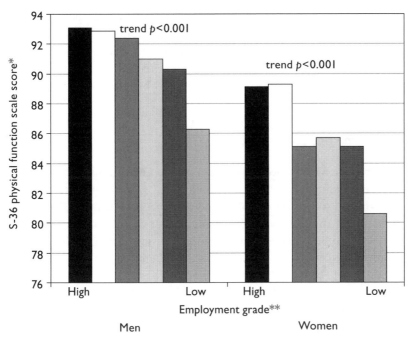

Notes: * SF-36 physical function score: 10-item self-reported scale (range 0–100, high score=high functioning) of health limitations affecting everyday physical activities including lifting, walking, bathing and dressing.
** Employment grade hierarchy from high to low: administrative 1, administrative 2, senior executive officer; higher executive officer, executive officer, clerical/office support.

Source: Hemingway et al (1997)

set point of these systems (Brunner, 1997, 2002). The allostatic load hypothesis (McEwen, 1998) is an important formulation of this concept, and relevant to CVD, cancer, infection, cognitive decline and other aspects of ageing. The price of adaptation to external and internal stress may be wear and tear on the organism, the result of chronic over- or under-activity of physiological systems to produce allostatic load. For instance, the endocrine system controlling blood glucose may be pushed towards diabetes.

The major systems receiving attention in psychobiological and cardiovascular behavioural research involve the sympathetic and parasympathetic branches of the autonomic nervous system, and stress hormones cortisol and catecholamines. Other neuroendocrine pathways are under study and may be equally relevant (Manuck et al, 2004). The activity of these autonomic systems is largely beyond conscious control, although training can effectively modify it. Manifestations include a heart rate rise in response to excitement and anxiety, and parauresis or 'bashful bladder syndrome', which interferes with attempts to urinate in the presence of others.

Evidence is accumulating that patterns of autonomic and neuroendocrine responsivity can alter functioning of homeostatic systems controlling the level CVD risk markers. Laboratory-based studies further show that short-term responses may differ according to social position, consistent with a conditioning effect (Steptoe et al, 2002). Such differences may contribute to development of social gradients in metabolic syndrome, raised levels of inflammatory markers and blood coagulation factors.

Metabolic syndrome and stress markers

Metabolic syndrome is a well-known precursor state to CHD. It is highly prevalent in US adults (Ford et al, 2002). Central, or abdominal, obesity predicts CHD in men and women and is linked with increased risk of type T diabetes. The other main components of the metabolic syndrome cluster of risk factors (impaired glucose tolerance, insulin resistance, raised blood pressure and lipid disturbances including high serum triglycerides and low HDL cholesterol) are each also associated with raised coronary risk.

We have shown previously that there is a social gradient in the metabolic syndrome in Whitehall II participants (Brunner et al, 1997). This raised the possibility that the social gradient in heart disease could in part be explained by metabolic syndrome, which we saw above to be the case. It also suggested that by analysing the upstream determinants of metabolic syndrome we might be able to demonstrate psychosocial effects on risk of CVD and diabetes. First, however, we wanted to see if there was biological evidence, from hormonal and other autonomic measures, that chronic stress might have a causal role in metabolic syndrome.

Our approach turned out to be fruitful (Brunner et al, 2002). We studied a randomly selected group of men who continued to be in civil service employment, attempting to ensure that the group contained sufficient individuals with metabolic syndrome. A nurse went to their workplaces and showed them how to collect a 24-hour urine sample during a working week. The protocol was organised so that neither nurse nor participant knew the exact nature of the study hypothesis or which of the participants had metabolic syndrome. The results were remarkably supportive of the stress hypothesis given that we found only 30 cases in the study of 183 men. Compared with the control group, metabolic syndrome cases had higher urinary cortisol and normetanephrine (metabolites of norepinephrine) outputs, higher heart rates and lower heart rate variability (the last two of these measurements were made at a research clinic visit). Low heart rate variability (HRV) is a risk factor for coronary disease.

These findings simultaneously linked the two major neuroendocrine stress axes and autonomic activity of the heart with metabolic syndrome. Heart rate variability was lower, indicating predominance of stimulatory sympathetic neural inputs to the heart and reduced heart rate-lowering vagal inputs. Psychosocial factors and health-related behaviours explained in part the neuroendocrine disturbances that accompanied the syndrome. This study provides suggestive evidence that chronic psychosocial stress might contribute to development of metabolic syndrome. Because it is cross-sectional, it does not prove that stress is a causal factor. Further prospective studies are needed to eliminate the possibility that the neuroendocrine alterations are produced by the syndrome, rather than contributing to its development.

These fascinating results encouraged us to conduct a larger study of heart rate variability in the Whitehall II cohort. We examined the interrelationships of HRV and metabolic syndrome with employment grade and psychosocial factors (Hemingway et al, 2005). Measurement of HRV was made by means of a five-minute electrocardiogram recording. Lower social position in the sample of 2,197 men was associated with higher heart rate and lower HRV. All five risk factor components of metabolic syndrome, and the factor itself, were associated with low HRV. In addition, the relationship between lower social position and higher risk of metabolic syndrome was mediated by HRV, behavioural factors and low job control. This larger study provided population evidence for the hypothesis that disturbances of the autonomic nervous system are involved in mediating the excess coronary risk associated with low social position. It is cross-sectional, however, and so can be criticised for not demonstrating causal sequence.

Work stress and metabolic syndrome

Cross-sectional studies have linked work stress with components of metabolic syndrome (Brunner et al, 1996; Siegrist and Peter, 1997; Peter et al, 1998; Cesana et al, 2003), but this association proved not to be consistent (Schnall and Landsbergis, 1994; Vrijkotte et al, 1999). The lack of longitudinal studies was an important gap in the evidence for a causal effect, and the accumulated data over seven phases and 15 years of Whitehall II provided an opportunity to carry out a study taking the duration of exposure to work stress into account. Repeated measurements of work stress over a person's career provide a more accurate representation of psychosocial stress exposure and its cumulative effect on health (Chandola et al, 2005). We analysed the association between four phases of work stress measurement and metabolic syndrome over 14 years of follow-up, testing the hypothesis that there is a dose–response association (see Figure 8.4).

The study proved to show a clear dose–response relationship (Chandola et al, 2006). Employees with chronic work stress on three or more occasions had over twice the odds of the syndrome compared to those reporting no episodes of work stress, after adjustment for age and employment grade, and those reporting intermediate exposure levels were at intermediate levels of risk. Work stress in this study was measured by the iso-strain model (Karasek and Theorell, 1990; Landsbergis et al, 1994). Iso-strain is present when job demands are high, job decision latitude is low and work social support is low (that is, where there is a lack of supportive co-workers or supervisors). Accumulation of exposure to work stress over the four measurement periods (phases 1, 2, 3 and 5) was measured by

Figure 8.4: Dose–response effect of work stress (iso-strain) on incident metabolic syndrome (Whitehall II Study)

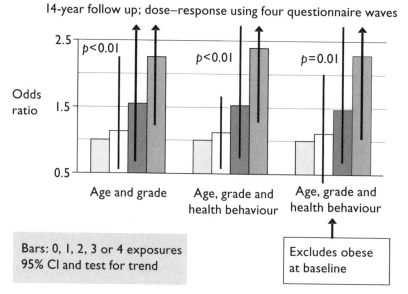

14-year follow up; dose–response using four questionnaire waves

Results are shown adjusted for age and grade (left hand panel); age, grade and health behaviours (centre panel); age, grade and health behaviours with exclusion of participants who were obese at study baseline (right hand panel).

Notes: x-axis labels show variables used in adjustment. Health behaviour = health behaviours over four exposure phases: current smoking, no daily fruit and vegetable consumption, heavy alcohol consumption drinkers (men > four units a day; women > three units a day), no exercise. Four bars show risk of metabolic syndrome respectively for no exposure (reference group), 1 exposure, 2 exposures, 3 or 4 exposures over the period of follow-up.

Source: Chandola et al (2006)

adding together the number of times the participant was exposed to iso-strain. The small degree to which the social gradient in metabolic syndrome is explained by taking account of exposure to iso-strain (approximately 6%) suggests that further refinement of our psychosocial exposure measure is needed. In contrast, the social gradient declined by 50% when iso-strain, health behaviours and obesity were entered into the model. Nevertheless there is a strong causal inference in this study. The prospective stress–metabolic syndrome relation was robust to adjustment for social position and variation in adverse health behaviours.

Organisational justice and heart disease

We have considered that there is a close relationship between work hierarchies and wider social structure. The qualities of the social order, in terms of the distribution of autonomy, reciprocity and justice, were seen above to have a firm basis in human preference, and potentially to provide a psychosocial explanation of the effects of relative inequality of health. In the work context, Whitehall II shows that perceived lack of reciprocity assessed by the effort–reward imbalance questionnaire is a predictor of CHD (Kuper et al, 2002) and that perception of organisational justice influences risk of disease (Kivimaki et al, 2005).

The organisational justice exposure measurement was based on five questionnaire items from the Karasek–Theorell job strain instrument (see Table 8.1) at phases 1 and 2 (1985–90).

Follow-up over nine years for CHD death, first non-fatal MI or definite angina occurring from phase 2 through 1999 was based on medical records. After adjustment for age and employment grade, employees who experienced a high level of justice at work had a lower risk of incident CHD than employees with a low or an intermediate level of justice (hazard ratio 0.65, 95% confidence interval 0.47–0.89). The size of the effect of organisational justice is remarkable. Although other psychosocial models of work stress (job strain and effort–reward imbalance) predicted CHD in these data, the level of justice remained an independent predictor of incident CHD after adjustment for these risk factors as well as employment grade and health behaviours.

Implications

The evidence presented in this overview chapter is drawn mainly from the Whitehall II Study. The occupational hierarchy is probably more rigid in the British civil service than in other large employers. This is not a weakness of the study, although it cannot be representative of the diversity of employment relations and conditions experienced in the workplace. It does, however, identify the health effects of working at different levels in a stratified organisation, and as such provides proof of principle. More speculatively, it may also identify some of the wider influences on health operating in the social hierarchy outside work, including social justice.

The policy implications of this body of work are far-reaching. In contrast to public health policy, which focuses on smoking and other health-related behaviours, measures are needed that address governance and organisational factors rather than the individual. Such measures would tackle mid-stream and upstream influences on health with the intention to reduce social inequalities in health. The Acheson Report in the UK reviewed the state of knowledge in the field of health inequalities for the incoming Labour government in 1997/98 and produced 39 recommendations in 13 broad groupings (Acheson, 1998). In the employment group, recommended policies were quantitative and qualitative in nature. They included improvement of employment opportunities, and investment in high-quality training for young and long-term unemployed people. Acheson proposed policies to improve the quality of work, and specifically to reduce psychosocial work hazards through reviews of management practices, aiming for increased levels of control, variety and use of skills in the workforce. The qualitative aspects of the recommendations have been taken up by the statutory occupational health agency, the Health and Safety Executive, through the introduction of voluntary management standards with accompanying guidelines on assessment of workplace psychosocial conditions.

Beyond the workplace, Acheson recommended policies that challenge the status quo at the national level. These encourage redistribution of material resources through alterations in taxation and social security benefits with a particular focus on women of childbearing age, young children and older people. The overall aim of such policies is to reduce the level of social inequality and to redistribute power and capability across the nation. It is ambitious but the evidence supports the view that population health, in the widest sense, will benefit.

References

Acheson, D. (1998) *Inequalities in health: Report of an independent inquiry*, London: HMSO.

Bajekal, M. (2005) 'Healthy life expectancy by area deprivation: magnitude and trends in England, 1994-1999', *Health Statistics Quarterly* 25: 18-27.

Brunner, E J. (1997) 'Socioeconomic determinants of health: stress and the biology of inequality', *British Medical Journal* 314: 1472-6.

Brunner, E.J. (2002) 'Stress mechanisms in coronary heart disease', in S.A. Stansfeld and M.G. Marmot (eds) *Stress and the heart: Psychosocial pathways to coronary heart disease*, London: BMJ Books: 181-99.

Brunner, E.J., Davey Smith, G., Marmot, M.G., Canner, R., Beksinska, M. and O'Brien, J. (1996) 'Childhood social circumstances and psychosocial and behavioural factors as determinants of plasma fibrinogen', *Lancet* 347: 1008-13.

Brunner, E.J., Hemingway, H, Walker, B.R., Page, M., Clarke, P., Juneja, M. et al (2002) 'Adrenocortical, autonomic, and inflammatory causes of the metabolic syndrome', *Circulation* 106: 2659-65.

Brunner, E.J., Marmot, M.G., Nanchahal, K., Shipley, M.J., Stansfeld, S.A., Juneja, M. et al (1997) 'Social inequality in coronary risk: central obesity and the metabolic syndrome. evidence from the WII study', *Diabetologia* 40(11): 1341-9.

Cesana, G., Sega, R., Ferrario, M., Chiodini, P., Corrao, G. and Mancia, G. (2003) 'Job strain and blood pressure in employed men and women: a pooled analysis of four Northern Italian population samples', *Psychosomatic Medicine* 65: 558-63.

Chandola, T. Brunner, E. and Marmot, M. (2006) 'Chronic stress at work and the metabolic syndrome: prospective study', *British Medical Journal* 332: 521-5.

Chandola, T., Siegrist, J. and Marmot, M. (2005) 'Do changes in effort–reward imbalance at work contribute to an explanation of the social gradient in angina?', *Occupational and Environmental Medicine* 62(4): 223-30.

Eagleton, T. (2003) *After theory*, New York: Basic Books.

Erikson, R. and Goldthorpe, J.H. (1992) *The constant flux*, Oxford: Clarendon Press.

Ford, E.S., Giles, W.H. and Dietz, W.H. (2002) 'Prevalence of the metabolic syndrome among US adults: findings from the Third National Health and Nutrition Examination Survey', *Journal of the American Medical Association* 287(3): 356-9.

Gilbody, S., Sheldon, T. and Wessely, S. (2006) 'Should we screen for depression?', *British Medical Journal* 332: 1027-30.

Hemingway, H., Shipley, M., Brunner, E., Britton, A., Malik, M. and Marmot, M.G. (2005) 'Does autonomic function link social position to coronary risk? The Whitehall II Study', *Circulation* 111: 3071-7.

Hemingway, H., Stafford, M., Stansfeld, S., Shipley, M.J. and Marmot, M. (1997) 'Is the SF-36 a valid measure of change in population health? Results from the Whitehall II Study', *British Medical Journal* 315(7118): 1273-9.

Kahneman, D., Diener, E. and Schwarz, N. (2003) *Well-being: The foundations of hedonic psychology*, New York: Russell Sage Foundation.

Karasek, R. and Theorell, T. (1990) *Healthy work: Stress, productivity, and the reconstruction of working life*, New York: Basic Books.

Kivimaki, M., Ferrie, J.E., Brunner, E.J., Head, J., Shipley, M.J., Vahtera, J. et al (2005) 'Justice at work and reduced risk of coronary heart disease among employees: the Whitehall II Study', *Archives of Internal Medicine* 165(19): 2245-51.

Kumari, M., Head, J. and Marmot, M. (2004) 'Prospective study of social and other risk factors for incidence of type 2 diabetes in the Whitehall II Study', *Archives of Internal Medicine* 164(17): 1873-80.

Kuper, H., Singh-Manoux, A., Siegrist, J. and Marmot, M. (2002) 'When reciprocity fails: effort–reward imbalance in relation to coronary heart disease and health functioning within the Whitehall II Study', *Occupational and Environmental Medicine* 59(11): 777-84.

Landsbergis, P.A., Schnall, P.L., Warren, K., Pickering, T.G. and Schwartz, J.E. (1994) 'Association between ambulatory blood pressure and alternative formulations of job strain', *Scandinavian Journal of Work and Environmental Health* 20: 349-63.

Layard, R. (2005) *Happiness: Lessons from a new science*, London: Penguin.

McEwen, B.S. (1998) 'Protective and damaging effects of stress mediators', *New England Journal of Medicine* 338: 171-9.

Manuck, S.B., Flory, J.D., Ferrell, R.E. and Muldoon, M.F. (2004) 'Socio-economic status covaries with central nervous system serotonergic responsivity as a function of allelic variation in the serotonin transporter gene-linked polymorphic region', *Psychoneuroendocrinology* 29: 651-68.

Marmot, M.G. and Brunner, E.J. (2005) 'Cohort profile: the Whitehall II Study', *International Journal of Epidemiology* 34(2): 251-6.

Marmot, M.G., Shipley, M.J. and Rose, G. (1984) 'Inequalities in death: specific explanations of a general pattern', *Lancet* 323: 1003-6.

Martikainen, P., Brunner, E. and Marmot, M. (2003) 'Socioeconomic differences in dietary patterns among middle-aged men and women', *Social Science and Medicine* 56: 1397-410.

Peter, R., Alfredsson, L., Hammar, N., Siegrist, J., Theorell, T. and Westerholm, P. (1998) 'High effort, low reward and cardiovascular risk factors in employed Swedish men and women: baseline results from the WOLF study', *Journal of Epidemiology and Community Health* 52: 540-7.

Rawls, J.A. (1971) *A theory of justice*, Cambridge, MA: Harvard University Press.

Rennie, K.L., McCarthy, N., Yazdgerdi, S., Marmot, M. and Brunner, E. (2003) 'Association of the metabolic syndrome with both vigorous and moderate physical activity', *International Journal of Epidemiology* 53: 600-6.

Schnall, P.L. and Landsbergis, P.A. (1994) 'Job strain and cardiovascular disease', *Annual Review of Public Health* 15: 381-411.

Siegrist, J. (1996) 'Adverse health effects of high-effort/low-reward conditions', *Journal of Occupational Health Psychology* 1: 27-41.

Siegrist, J. and Peter, R. (1997) 'Chronic work stress is associated with atherogenic lipids and elevated fibrinogen in middle-aged men', *Journal of Internal Medicine* 242(2): 149-56.

Stansfeld, S.A., Head, J., Fuhrer, R., Wardle, J. and Cattell, V. (2003) 'Social inequalities in depressive symptoms and physical functioning in the Whitehall II Study: exploring a common cause explanation', *Journal of Epidemiology and Community Health* 57: 361-7.

Steptoe, A., Feldman, P.J., Kunz, S., Owen, N., Willemsen, G. and Marmot, M. (2002) 'Stress responsivity and socioeconomic status: a mechanism for increased cardiovascular risk?', *European Heart Journal* 23: 1757-63.

Theorell, T. and Floderus-Myrhed, B. (1977) '"Workload" and risk of myocardial infarction: a prospective psychosocial analysis', *International Journal of Epidemiology* 6: 17-21.

Vrijkotte, T.G.M., van Doornen, L.J.P. and De Geus, E.J.C. (1999) 'Work stress and metabolic and hemostatic risk factors', *Psychosomatic Medicine* 61: 796-805.

NINE

Inequality, psychosocial health and societal health: a model of inter-group conflict

Siddharth Chandra

Introduction

The aim of this chapter is to present a model that links inequality with psychosocial health, and psychosocial health with group violence. In the process, I explore linkages between identity, inequality and the behaviour of groups using models and concepts from psychology, politics, sociology, economics and demography. At a variety of levels, these linkages can be thought of as driving a major public health outcome, namely violence.

Over the past two decades, a large literature has developed, which identifies violence as a public health problem. This literature has emphasised individual acts of violence that have a relatively high degree of prevalence in the US (Rosenberg and Fenley, 1991; Koop, 1992; Rosenberg, 1992; Krug et al, 2002). A number of studies on how to manage the problem, and specifically how to prevent acts of violence (Mercy and O'Carroll, 1988; Mercy et al, 1993; Saltzman et al, 2000), parallel the work that casts violence as a public health problem. If individual acts of violence spread out across time are a chronic public health problem, then it follows logically that a large number of interconnected acts of violence, occurring over a short period of time, should be considered an acute public health problem. Indeed, the public health literature already acknowledges ethnic violence as one form of the violence that the public health community needs to address (Foege et al, 1995). Hence, studying such violence with a view to understanding its causes and the conditions under which the likelihood of such acts can be reduced should form an important focus within the field of public health policy. The motivation for this chapter is to begin to study one such phenomenon.

Specifically, I use an existing model of individual identity, which makes predictions about behavioural outcomes at the individual level. In this model, inequality plays an instrumental role in shaping individual identity. Following this, I aggregate up from the individual to the group to demonstrate implications of this model for group behaviour. The implicit argument is that certain types of group behaviour resulting from inequality are symptomatic of ill-health at the individual level. This psychosocial model is linked to demographic change to demonstrate the kinds of outcomes that can occur at the aggregate level. These population-level outcomes can also be viewed as a form of societal ill-health.

Briefly, the causal model is depicted in Figure 9.1. Inequality drives identity formation and demographic change. Specifically, demographic change is driven by differential population growth across identity groups. Coupled with demographic change, identity formation drives the need for political change, and in particular a demand for the transfer of power across identity groups. Political regimes, democratic or non-democratic, determine the nature of the resolution of this demand, which can be accompanied by large-scale violence.

The emphasis in this chapter is on those portions of the model that are new to the literature. Where the model relies on existing bodies of knowledge, reference is made to the literature in the abbreviated discussion. The conclusion is that, to the extent that inequality can result in the polarisation of society on the lines of characteristics that shape identity and behaviour, it can drive this kind of social (and individual) ill-health. Further, the outcomes of this polarisation can have more direct consequences for health. Finally, political institutions can play a crucial role in reducing or eliminating some of the potentially devastating outcomes of inequality and the polarisation it can cause.

Self-theory and identity: psychosocial foundations

This chapter draws on the literature on self-theory, an area of enquiry within social psychology that seeks to explain the processes that give rise to the notion of the self (Markus and Cross, 1990; Robins et al, 1999; Tessor et al, 2000; Andersen and Chen, 2002; Leary and Tangney, 2003). An understanding of these processes

Figure 9.1: Schematic of the model

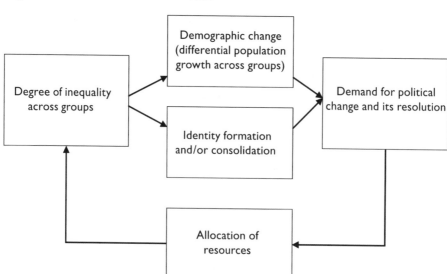

can shed light on such individual-level phenomena as mood, self-esteem and, more broadly, behaviour (Cervone and Mischel, 2002). In the present context, the attraction of this body of literature is its ability to interface with the study of identity formation, which often goes hand in hand with inequality, and can lead to situations of individual and social ill-health (Chandra and Williams-Foster, 2004). Specifically, I use a portfolio-theoretic model (Chandra and Shadel, 2007) of the self to demonstrate the implications of inequality for such outcomes. This section summarises the portfolio-theoretic model of the self with a view to tying it to the analysis of the issue at hand, namely violence between different identity groups.

In the portfolio-theoretic model, the self is constructed from an underlying finite universe of 'self-attributes'. Self-attributes are attributes that are descriptive of the self. Examples of self-attributes include 'aggressive', 'sociable' and 'independent'. A self-attribute may have a negative or a positive valence, meaning that the attribute may contribute negatively or positively to an individual-level outcome of interest such as mood. At any given time, an individual may be more or less 'schematic' on any given self-attribute. The concept of schematicity combines the extent to which a particular self-attribute is important to and descriptive of the self at any given time. Schematicity over a self-attribute can vary over time, depending on the situational context of the individual. Over time, therefore, and depending on the specific situation and context, an individual may be schematic over differing combinations of self-attributes, leading to different outcomes of mood and behaviour. An understanding of how self-attributes are organised to produce these individual-level outcomes is, therefore, crucial.

The portfolio-theoretic model of the self views the self as a portfolio of self-attributes. The model is operationally very similar to the model of an asset portfolio in finance (Markowitz, 1952, 1956, 1959; Hester and Tobin, 1967; Elton and Gruber, 1991). A well-known class of asset portfolio is the mutual fund. Investors invest in mutual funds in order to diversify their risk, or reduce the variability of returns that they will receive on their investment. Diversification is possible precisely because, in any given mutual fund, some stocks are likely to rise in value to counter the effects of declines in the value of other stocks. As a consequence, it is highly unlikely that the value of the mutual fund, whose fortunes are tied to the fortunes of a diverse mix of companies, will fluctuate as much as that of a single stock, whose value is tied to the fortunes of a single company. Diversification of a portfolio is typically achieved by spreading the investment relatively equally across a large number of assets, each of which has a pattern of returns that is not very highly correlated with those of the other assets in the portfolio.

A key outcome of the portfolio-theoretic model of the self is the analogous prediction that, the more the self-concept is like a well-diversified mutual fund (and less like a stock), the greater is the stability in individual-level outcomes to which the structure gives rise. In short, a self-concept that is very heavily weighted (in the sense of the individual tending to be highly schematic) on one or a few similarly valenced self-attributes whose schematicities tend to move together, the more instability one is likely to observe with respect to the mood and behaviour of the individual. Conversely, a self-concept that is equally or similarly weighted (again in the sense of the individual tending to be schematic) on a large number of self-attributes whose valences tend to buffer one another, the more stability one is likely to observe with respect to the mood and behaviour of the individual. This prediction has recently been validated for mood in an empirical study (Chandra and Shadel, 2007).

Inequality, relative deprivation and identity: the interplay of social context and identity

A second body of literature on which this chapter draws lies in an area of overlap between psychology, sociology and political science. Inequality has long been tied to the notion of relative deprivation, a phenomenon that occurs at the level of the individual. Relative deprivation is said to occur when an individual feels that they are not receiving what they deserve from society (Gurr, 1970). Most people feel relatively deprived at one point or another in their lives. This is a natural and common phenomenon. We tend to have an idea of our ability and value, and we tend to benchmark what we deserve on our observations of the benefits other people with differing abilities receive from society. Relative deprivation occurs when what we receive, typically measured by income, falls short of our assessment, based on our observations of other people, of what we should be receiving. Often, it takes the perception of a pattern, rather than an individual (random) instance, to create feelings of relative deprivation among people. For an example of the role of relative deprivation in protest movements, see Chandra and Williams-Foster (2005).

Once it has set in, however, relative deprivation can have profound consequences for identity. If, in addition to the systematic observation that the individual is receiving less than they deserve from society, the individual also observes that a similar form of deprivation is incident on other members of society who share a certain characteristic (such as race), the identity of the individual may begin to transform into one that is more and more similar to those of the other 'similar' individuals. There are a variety of reasons for this, including the need to find an explanation for a perceived injustice. The result of this dynamic is the concentrating of the self-concept around a set of self-attributes that define a notion of identification with the broader 'wronged' group.

This concentrating of the self-concept around a specific set of self-attributes can have a reinforcing effect on the sense of relative deprivation. The more the self-concept shares with those of the other members of the group, the more attuned the individual is to inequalities between members of the group and society in general. The consequence of this mutually reinforcing dynamic between a sense of relative deprivation and the transformation of the identity is the creation of an individual or group of individuals that regards themselves as separate from the rest of society.

Why is relative deprivation such a powerful driver of this polarisation? Research has shown that increments in well-being add much less to our happiness than decreases in well-being take away from it. People tend to be 'loss averse', and relative deprivation essentially involves a sense of loss over what should have been (Kahneman and Tversky, 1979). While individuals have various means of adapting to such feelings, a common one is to try to find an explanation for the situation. In the case of relative deprivation, this may result in a downward adjustment of the individual's sense of self-worth. Alternatively, the individual may blame it on socioeconomic rigidities beyond their control, as a consequence of which the outcome is inherently unjust. When this occurs, the individual may unite with other members of the wronged group in order to seek redress.

A common way in which individuals or groups of similar (in the sense of the make-up of the self-concept) individuals cope with relative deprivation is to ascribe the cause to socioeconomic rigidities. If the incidence of relative deprivation across a population of individuals systematically coincides with a recognisable aspect of identity, then society is vulnerable to polarisation. Note that, in the context of the portfolio-theoretic model of the self described above, an 'aspect' of identity may be a single self-attribute or a cluster of self-attributes that hang together in a contextually meaningful way. Thus, a specific pattern of schematicity over a subset of the self-attribute universe may define belonging to a particular ethnic, religious, linguistic, racial or national group. To the extent that relative deprivation may occur systematically across individuals who are very similar in a particular aspect of their identity, the situation may create a self-reinforcing dynamic. In other words, there is a socioeconomic rigidity born out of some real or perceived difference between people, which reinforces the difference, which reinforces the cause and so forth. It is not hard to see how groups can become boxed into a situation of relative deprivation, leading, in the longer term, to pressures for drastic social change. The aim of this chapter is to explore, using concepts from demography, a special case of this dynamic.

The association between per-capita income and fertility is established to the point that economists and historians now take it as a given in constructing models of economic growth and population change (see, for example, de la Croix and Doepke, 2003). Economists and demographers have constructed various models explaining this association. A well-known model is the Becker-Murphy model (Becker et al, 1990) in which parents with high levels of human capital (education) tend to prefer to have children with high levels of human capital. Hence, they invest more resources in smaller numbers of children, in contrast with parents with lower levels of human capital, who invest their resources in larger numbers of children with lower per-capita human capital input. Because high human capital is highly correlated with high income, this translates into a relationship between levels of income and fertility.

This notion ties neatly into situations in which there are two identity groups with vastly differing levels of per-capita income. Specifically, it predicts that the poorer group will experience a high rate of population growth (via high fertility) relative to the wealthier group. Depending on the initial population breakdown and the distribution of political power, sustained differentials in the rate of population growth across identity groups can have serious implications for social harmony and can set the stage for inter-group conflict and, perhaps, even violence (Strand and Urdal (2005). In the following section, I present a model that ties together the concepts presented above and generates predictions for the occurrence of inter-group violence.

A model of inequality, relative deprivation, demographic change and sociopolitical outcomes

In the specific model in this chapter I make the following simplifying assumptions:

(1) There are two identifiable and distinguishable groups in society. These may be religious sects, racial groups, linguistic groups or groups defined on the basis of some other commonly observed social fault line.
(2) The individuals belonging to one group are deprived relative to the individuals in the other group in terms of per-capita income, wealth or well-being. Individuals belonging to the systematically deprived group feel a sense of relative deprivation and they are prepared to act to eliminate this inequality.
(3) Economic resources, which determine the income, wealth or well-being of the individuals in the groups, are allocated depending on the degree of control that each group exercises on the political system.
(4) Group membership cannot change over time, and a person born of parents in one group is a member of that group for life.
(5) In keeping with established economic phenomena, the poor group has a higher rate of population growth than the relatively wealthy group.

To these assumptions I add three initial conditions:

(6) Initially, the poor group is small in terms of the number of members relative to the wealthy group.
(7) Initially, political power rests in the hands of the larger and wealthier group.
(8) The political institutions in society are democratic in the sense that the political power of each group is proportional to the fraction of people belonging to that group in the population. As the composition of the population varies, so too does the political power of each group.

In combination with the three initial conditions (6)–(8), the five assumptions (1)–(5) lead to an interesting outcome. Over time, because the poorer group is growing more rapidly in numbers than the relatively wealthy group, it will become the majority. Because it is a relatively deprived majority that is willing to act to do away with systematic inequity, the pressure for socioeconomic change will build. The ultimate outcome in society will be a gradual move over from a situation in which the original relatively wealthy majority gradually becomes a relatively less wealthy minority. The degree to which these socioeconomic changes lag behind the transfer of political power will determine the degree to which the once-wealthy majority becomes a relatively deprived minority. At this point, the tables will have turned, and the same dynamic as the one described above will occur, but in reverse. Thus, we have a cyclical pattern of alternating relative deprivation for the two groups in society.

The linkages described above can be demonstrated using a very simple and specific quantitative model. The model works as follows. The population consists of two identifiable groups. In year 1, one group has a population of 1,000 and the second group has a population of 100. For simplicity, I assume that, after attaining adulthood, each person produces the same amount of value for society, and is compensated accordingly. Therefore, the total income accruing to society is assumed to be equal to the total population in society, but with a lag. The logic of the lag is the idea that a person becomes economically active some years after they are born. By the time a given cohort of the population becomes economically active, then, the total population in society will have grown in size. The per-capita income for each group is the total income for the group divided by the population of that group. Hence, if a group is growing rapidly in size, the difference between the total population of that group (that is, productive and non-productive people) will be large, and the per-capita income of that group will be low compared to a group that is growing more slowly.

The rate of population growth for each group is modelled to be decreasing in the per-capita income of the group. This is in line with the assumption that fertility and therefore population growth are negatively related with income. The rate of population growth for each group is also modelled to be decreasing in a time-varying parameter that is the reciprocal of total income in the economy per person in the group. This time-varying parameter ensures that, if the income of the other group is significantly higher than the income in the reference group, then the reference group, being relatively deprived, will have a higher population growth rate. In other words, the higher the per-capita income of a group, the lower the population growth, and the lower the per-capita income relative to that of the other group, the more rapidly population grows.

Figures 9.2 and 9.3 demonstrate what happens in this model. If the time lag between population growth and economic maturity is small, say five time periods, then the system quickly equilibrates in the sense that the two subpopulations equalise and grow at equal rates (Figure 9.2). If the time lag between population growth and economic maturity is large, say 50 time periods, then the system is never in equilibrium if we define an equilibrium as equal populations for each group, and we have a pattern of fluctuating majority for the two groups (see Figure 9.3).

While the model presented here is very simple and specific, it is possible to relax some of the more stringent assumptions and still yield the kinds of equilibria displayed in Figures 9.2 and 9.3.

Figure 9.2: Log of population over time

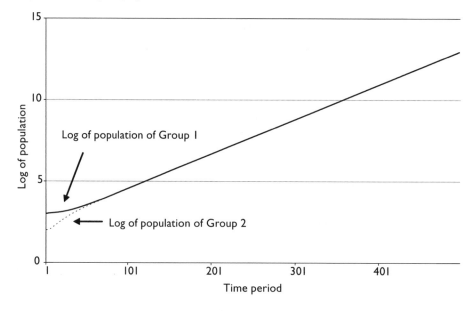

Figure 9.3: Log of population over time

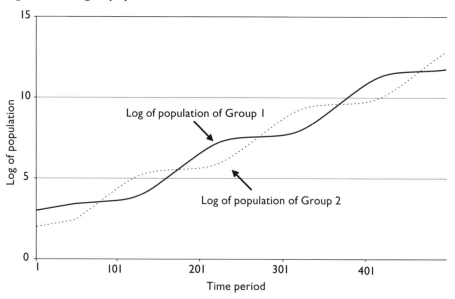

If we change initial condition (7) to:

(7a) The political institutions in society are strongly authoritarian, with the authoritarian ruler belonging to and favouring the initially wealthy majority.

then a remarkable and disturbing set of outcomes becomes possible. The notable difference between this situation and the earlier model is the absence of the democratic institutions that act as a pressure valve for the elimination of the systematic inequalities in society. In this case, pressure for change will continue to build up well beyond the point that the once-poor and relatively deprived minority has become the majority. This is a dangerous situation that can result in political upheaval accompanied, perhaps, by violence. If the violence does not result in some drastic change in demography (which can reduce or temporarily eliminate the pressure for change through genocide, for example), only the installation of a new system, be it authoritarian with a leader favourable to the new and still relatively deprived majority, or democratic, will serve to reduce the pressure that has built up for change.

Summary and evaluation of the model

The model presented in this chapter has several strengths and weaknesses. It is one of the first of its kind in that it models linkages between individual psychology, economic inequality, demography and politics. It uses some well-established facts and recent research findings to produce empirically testable predictions. Unlike a variety of models in psychology and political science, which have a short-term (single-generation) focus, it is a multigenerational model. Because of the broad scope of the model, it also has many weaknesses. For example, the multigenerational nature of the model is as much a weakness as it is a strength. Because of the duration necessary for the dynamics of the model to have an influence on outcomes, it is likely that, in many cases, events exogenous to the model will intervene to create effects that may disguise or complicate the processes in the model. A second area of weakness is the general case in which there are more than two groups, making for more complicated interactions between groups, such as coalitional politics. The less parsimonious and more complex a model becomes, however, the greater is its ability to explain a specific outcome, but the less generalisable is the model.

These issues suggest a number of future directions for research on the links between inequality, psychosocial ill-health, political demography and violence on the lines suggested above. The broader class of models to which the specific model of this chapter belongs is versatile. It can admit multiple groups, with the attendant issues of coalition-building that the analysis of such a model might entail. It can allow for demographic change through migration, necessitating the inclusion of concepts of the drivers of migration and the political activity of migrants. It can capture other forms of demographic change, such as those caused by disease or war, which may modify the dynamics of the simple scenario presented above. Hence, at the level of formal model-building, the future agenda is the creation of a set of formal models that covers more thoroughly the space defined by this class of models.

A second direction for future research is the empirical validation of the above models. Simply put, do we observe the kinds of dynamics that the models predict? While this line of enquiry is fraught with challenges, including the possible absence of quality demographic and economic data going back more than a few generations and the occurrence of various 'shocks', including wars and changes in national boundaries, it would nevertheless be instructive to try to identify cases in which variants of the models have some explanatory power, and others in which the models fail. This exercise could lead to the modification or refinement of the basic ideas that this study proposes. At the very least, it would illuminate the utility of this theoretical line of thinking.

A third direction for future research is the role of public policy in preventing or mitigating the effects of demographically driven inter-group violence. What role should the government play to prevent such violence from occurring? Should it, as has been the case in a number of countries, design policies to alter differential rates of population growth so as to maintain a demographic status quo, eliminating the build-up of pressure for political change? Or, should it allow differential rates of population growth, allowing for the possibility of political upheaval, and preparing instead to manage the consequences of this upheaval?

This leads to the fourth and final direction for future research stemming from this model. What are the implications of this body of theory for public health policy? How should societies possessing the preconditions for inter-group conflict invest in a public health infrastructure to manage the outcomes of such conflict? What kinds of interventions at the psychosocial level reduce the likelihood of such outcomes? What role can education play in mitigating some of the psychosocial ill-health that may develop from demographic change in the presence of relative deprivation?

Conclusion

In line with the recent literature in public health, this chapter has taken the approach that violence is a form of public ill-health (Foege et al, 1995). Therefore, it is imperative that the public health community studies the forms and causes of violence in an effort to reduce its prevalence, if not eliminate it. The goal of this chapter was to study inter-group violence, with a view to understanding some of its causes and the mechanisms that may give rise to it.

At the base of inter-group violence lie concepts of identity and polarisation, both of which can and often are related to inequality in society. In order to model inter-group violence, therefore, I use an existing model of individual identity, which makes predictions about behavioural outcomes at the individual level. In this model, inequality plays an instrumental role in shaping individual identity. Following this, I aggregate up from the individual to the group to demonstrate implications of this model for group behaviour. The implicit argument is that certain types of group behaviour resulting from inequality are symptomatic of ill-health at the individual level. This psychosocial model is linked to demographic change to demonstrate the kinds of outcomes, including inter-group violence, that can occur at the aggregate level. As a large body of work in the public health literature rightly argues, these population-level outcomes can also be viewed as a form of societal ill-health, and one that is as broad in its scope as it is profound in its effects on large numbers of people.

In the past, most societies dealt with the public health repercussions of inequality and demographic change in a reactive manner. Usually, it is only after the violence has erupted that governments have mobilised to reduce its occurrence and the sometimes horrible public health outcomes that it brings. Thinking about such violence as a public health issue will help to frame the problem in a proactive and potentially much more constructive manner. Just as some pathogen-borne epidemics can be prevented with programmes of biological immunisation, so can public health and other authorities take a proactive approach to the prevention of inter-group violence. To the extent that concepts from psychology, demography, sociology and political science can inform the mechanisms that may predispose individuals and groups to this form of violence, it is imperative that these concepts be brought into the discourse on the role of public health policy in mitigating inter-group violence.

References

Andersen, S. M. and Chen, S. (2002) 'The relational self: an interpersonal social-cognitive theory', *Psychological-Review* 109: 619-45.

Becker, G.S., Murphy, K.M. and Tamura, R. (1990) 'Human capital, fertility, and economic growth', *Journal of Political Economy* 98 (Suppl 5): 12.

Cervone, D. and Mischel, W. (2002) 'Personality science', in D. Cervone and W. Mischel (eds) *Advances in personality science*, New York: Guilford Press: 1-26.

Chandra, S. and Shadel, W.G. (2007) 'Crossing disciplinary boundaries: applying portfolio theory from the field of finance to extend self-schema theory from the field of personality', *Journal of Research in Personality*, 41(2): 346-73.

Chandra, S. and Williams-Foster, A. (2005) 'The "revolution of rising expectations", relative deprivation and the urban social disorders of the 1960s: evidence from state-level data', *Social Science History*, 29(2): 299-332.

de la Croix, D. and Doepke, M. (2003) 'Inequality and growth: why differential fertility matters', *American Economic Review* 93(4): 1091-113.

Foege, W. H., Rosenberg, M.L. and Mercy, J.A. (1995) 'Public health and violence prevention', *Current Issues in Public Health* 1: 2-9.

Elton, E.J. and Gruber, M.J. (1991) *Modern portfolio theory and investment analysis*, New York: Wiley.

Gurr, T.R. (1970) *Why men rebel*, Princeton, NJ: Princeton University Press.

Hester, D.D. and Tobin, J. (eds) (1967) *Risk aversion and portfolio choice*, Monograph 19 of the Cowles Foundation for Research in Economics at Yale University, New York: John Wiley.

Kahneman, D. and Tversky, A. (1979) 'Prospect theory: an analysis of decision under risk', *Econometrica*, 47: 263–91.

Koop, C. (1992) 'Violence in America: a public health emergency. Time to bite the bullet back', *The Journal of the American Medical Association* 267(22): 3075.

Krug, E., Mercy, J., Dahlberg, L. and Zwi, A. (2002) 'The World Report on Violence and Health', *The Lancet*, 360(9339): 1083–8.

Leary, M.P. and Tangney, J.P. (2003) *Handbook of self and identity*, New York: Guilford Press.

Markowitz, H.M. (1952) 'Portfolio selection', *Journal of Finance* 7: 77-91.

Markowitz, H.M. (1956) 'The optimization of a quadratic function subject to linear constraints', *Naval Research Logistics Quarterly* 111: 111-33.

Markowitz, H.M. (1959) *Portfolio selection: Efficient diversification of investments*, Monograph 16 of the Cowles Foundation for Research in Economics at Yale University, New York: John Wiley.

Markus, H. and Cross, S. (1990) 'The interpersonal self', in L.A. Pervin (ed) *Handbook of personality: Theory and research*, New York, NY: Guilford Press: 576-608.

Mercy, J. A. and O'Carroll, P.W. (1988) 'New directions in violence prediction: the public health arena', *Violence and Victims* 3(4): 285-301.

Mercy, J.A., Rosenberg, M.L., Powell, K.E., Broome, C.V. and Roper, W.L. (1993) 'Public health policy for preventing violence', *Health Affairs* 12(4): 7-29.

Robins, R.W., Norem, J.K. and Cheek, J.M. (1999) 'Naturalizing the self', in L.A. Pervin and O.P. John (eds) *Handbook of personality: Theory and research* (2nd edition), New York, NY: Guilford Press: 443-77.

Rosenberg, M.L. (1992) 'Let's be clear. violence is a public health problem', *The Journal of the American Medical Association* 267(22): 3071.

Rosenberg, M.L. and Fenley, M.A. (1991) *Violence in America: A public health approach*, Oxford: Oxford University Press.

Saltzman, L.E., Green, Y.T., Marks, J.S. and Thacker, S.B. (2000) 'Violence against women as a public health issue: comments from the CDC', *American Journal of Preventative Medicine* 19(4): 325-9.

Strand, H. and Urdal, H. (2005) 'Differential growth, political instability and violent conflict', Presented at the 46th Annual Convention of the International Studies Association, Honolulu, HI, 1-5 March.

Tessor, A., Felson, R.B. and Suls, J.M. (2000) *Psychological perspectives on self and identity*, Washington, DC: American Psychological Association.

TEN

The social epidemiology of population health during the time of transition from communism in Central and Eastern Europe

Arjumand Siddiqi, Martin Bobak and Clyde Hertzman

Introduction

The present study offers a social epidemiological perspective on population health in Central and Eastern Europe (CEE) following the major societal transition there in the late 1980s and early 1990s. During this time, in much of CEE, a change of guard occurred from Soviet-style communist regimes to equally 'fundamentalist' capitalist (free-market) economic approaches; a phenomenon described as 'shock therapy' that was marked by a breakdown in the trade relationships among the Warsaw Pact countries, rapid economic decline and high rates of unemployment and inflation (Sachs, 1994; Brainerd, 1997; Klein and Pomer, 2001).

This was also a period of rapid political change. Although the end of the Soviet era brought with it free speech and a system of parliamentary democracy, instability was rampant in the region, with democracy-watchers concerned that electoral patterns revealed the fragility of the reform process (United Nations Development Programme, 1996). In psychosocial terms, CEE showed a low prevalence of post-material attitudes (for example, concern for 'higher-order' values such as free speech and democracy, compared with more 'basic' concerns such as price inflation and maintenance of basic order in society), consistent with the pattern observed in poor countries (Abramson and Inglehart, 1995).

Population health statistics suggest that during the first four years of the transition period, there were dramatic increases in mortality among males and females of working age. Among males aged 30–49, mortality rose as much as 70-80% in Russia, 30–50% in Ukraine and 10–20% in Bulgaria, Hungary and Romania. Among females, mortality in the same age range rose 30–60% in Russia, 20–30% in Ukraine and more modestly in Bulgaria, Hungary and Romania (UNICEF, 1994).

The conditions leading to this mortality increase were primarily cardiovascular and external causes of death (UNICEF, 1994). However, these were also the most prevalent conditions in working-age persons at the beginning of the transition period; mortality due to these two causes was increasing even before the end of the Soviet period. This chapter suggests, then, that explaining the health crisis in CEE must go beyond understanding the determinants of these conditions, and address the factors that created general risk of mortality, in particular among the working-age population. The working premise is that the vulnerability in this group was general: that it was a crisis in health status that simply expressed itself through the principal causes of mortality for its age group.

This study therefore utilises 'perceived overall health' as the primary outcome of interest. In the absence of individual-level data on cardiovascular disease and external causes of death, perceived health provides an indication of general health status in this population. Further, self-rated health is highly correlated with clinical manifestations of health and illness and with mortality (Bobak et al, in press). We therefore submit that this health metric sheds much-needed light on the declines in population health in CEE during this time.

It is argued here that the transformations in CEE created conditions of loss of control over life, economic deprivation and social isolation, which, in turn, undermined the health status of the population. This disproportionately affected the male working-age population because their particular work and family support roles make them most vulnerable to socioeconomic shocks, especially when these shocks could not be buffered by a well-functioning state or civil society. Methodological approaches to studying such societal-level phenomena are also discussed, in particular with regard to the merits of cross-national and historical perspectives.

The bullseye model of social determinants of health

The present study uses the 'bullseye' model to investigate societal determinants of health. The model is the result of observations derived from the social epidemiological literature. The model suggests that the socioeconomic and psychological determinants of health function at three levels of aggregation in society. At the highest level of aggregation are the socioeconomic characteristics of the nation, such as the level and distribution of income and wealth created in the marketplace and the degree to which resulting inequalities are buffered by taxes, transfers and the redistributive characteristics of social programmes (Wilkinson, 1996; Ross et al, 2000). At the intermediate level of aggregation, there is civil society; that is, those features of social organisation such as institutional responsiveness, social trust, social cohesion and access to social goods (such as healthcare and education) that may either exacerbate or buffer the stresses of the broader socioeconomic environment and of daily existence generally (Putnam, 1993; Rose, 1995a; Kawachi et al, 1997). Finally, at the 'micro' level, there is the intimate realm of the family: its economic circumstances and the personal support network (Berkman and Glass, 2000).

The bullseye model summarises these relationships in the following manner. It represents societies by three concentric circles that stand for the clusters of determinants of health at the three levels of social aggregation described earlier (Figure 10.1). In addition, the central role of the individual lifecourse is represented by an arrow, piercing the bullseye. This is meant to create the impression of population health as an 'emergent function' of the lifelong interplay between material, behavioural, cognitive and emotional coping opportunities and vulnerabilities of *developing* individuals in the population, on the one hand, and the socioeconomic and psychological conditions as they present themselves at the intimate, civic and state level, on the other. That is, socioeconomic and psychological conditions change individuals in a variety of ways that affect their health prospects and, in turn, individuals and groups of individuals transform society through their responses to the environments in which they grow up, live, and work.

In some respects, this model is analogous to the Dahlgren and Whitehead (1991) framework. Both models describe the influence of various socioeconomic conditions on health outcomes, but the levels of aggregation are different in each. Also, the role of civil society is incorporated in the bullseye model, but not explicated in the Dahlgren and Whitehead framework. Finally, through its inclusion of the lifecourse perspective, the bullseye model addresses temporal aspects of the association between social conditions and subsequent health outcomes.

The model is not meant to imply that everyone in society responds equally to each determinant of health. Rather, combinations of factors that support or undermine health may differ for different individuals and populations. For example, we hypothesise gender differences in 'exposure' and 'response' to determinants of health: differences in gender roles may make different aspects of the lifecourse

Figure 10.1: Bullseye model of societal determinants of health

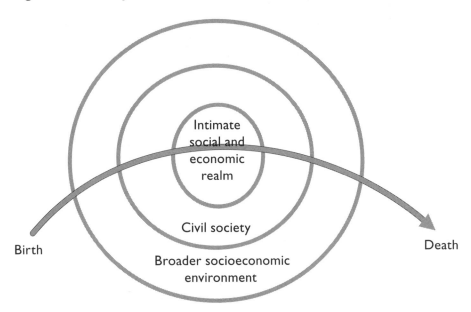

and environment more or less important, or there may be differential valuation, by gender, of the meaningfulness of different facets of the socioeconomic and psychological environment.

Testing the bullseye model of health during the transition period in CEE

This study applied the bullseye model to understanding the drastic increase in working-age mortality in CEE during the post-communist transition period. Due to limitations of data availability, empirical tests of the inner-most concentric circle of the model (representing individual social and economic circumstances) were performed using data from Russia only. For the middle circle, representing civil society, data were derived from Russia as well as several other CEE nations.

Due to a lack of multilevel data, the effects of the outer socioeconomic environment could not be empirically assessed in relation to individual self-rated health. With a multilevel data structure, testing a research hypothesis of the present type would require information on individuals that are in turn nested in nations – and enough nations to provide the power to test national-level hypotheses at that. Instead, descriptive analysis of this outermost circle of the bullseye model was carried out using data from a variety of CEE nations.

Multilevel versus ecologic data for studying societal conditions as determinants of health

In general, the capacity of researchers to conduct rigorous empirical investigations of the influence of the national sphere on individual health is hampered by a lack of availability of multilevel data. As such, questions of this nature are underinvestigated, despite their obvious importance. We suggest here that valuable insights are provided by using available ecologic data on socioeconomic factors occurring at the national level to describe the context in which associations between individual health and more micro-level determinants manifest.

At the very least, understandings of social and economic circumstances of a nation provide a basis for speculation and hypothesis generation. However, it is not only as a lesser substitute for multilevel data that marrying ecologic-level information with individual level data becomes useful. As discussed elsewhere, ecologic-level data also provide an opportunity for cross-national and historical comparisons that shed new light on the effects of socioeconomic conditions on health; a perspective that is difficult to replicate with multilevel data structures (Siddiqi and Hertzman, 2007).

To date, the preponderance of evidence regarding societal influences on population health has been acquired across relatively short timescales, largely confined to processes that unfold within an individual lifetime. This creates a problem that goes beyond the relative scientific merit of cross-sectional versus longitudinal research. The issue at hand is the timeframe of interest in which causal influences and their resultant health outcomes unfold at the level of society.

The timescale over which a society develops (or destroys) health-enhancing infrastructure and social safety-net functions may be quite long (Siddiqi and Hertzman, 2007).

On the other hand, the ways in which these societal phenomena manifest in the daily lives of individuals can only be effectively understood using individual-level data. The following analysis therefore lends support to the combined use of individual-level data to draw empirical associations, and societal-level data in both historical and cross-national perspective, to provide the context in which to understand more micro-level analyses.

Methods

Data sources and sample

To test the effects of individual-level social and economic factors, data from the sixth New Russia Barometer Survey were used. This survey was carried out after the presidential elections of 1996. The information was collected by the Russian Centre of Public Opinion Research (VCIOM) during a one-week period in July of that year. A multi-stage sample of the Russian population aged 18 years and over was selected. The Russian Federation was first stratified into 22 regions, then into urban and rural areas, and then, for rural areas, into regional centres and other towns. Within this framework, 69 urban and rural settlements were randomly drawn. In each settlement, households were listed by address, an address was selected randomly as the starting point and 161 interviewers were instructed to seek an interview at every n-th house. At each address the interviewer asked for a respondent matching an age by gender by education grid. Face-to-face interviews were conducted.

Of 3,379 households with someone at home, in 965 cases no one met the requirements of the age–sex–education grid. Of the 2,414 remaining households, in 470 (20%) the interview was refused, in 271 (11%) the door was not answered, in 63 (3%) the identified individual was unable to answer and 11 interviews (0.4%) were interrupted and therefore terminated early. The 1,599 completed interviews represent a final response rate of 66%, and correspond well with the age, sex and education distribution of the Russian population. In this chapter, the analyses are restricted to those aged 35 and over (n=1,138).

To measure civil society, data from the Centre for Public Policy Studies at the University of Strathclyde, Glasgow, Scotland were used. In addition, the Russia Barometer Survey provided a measure of individuals' 'view on civil society'. To measure the broader socioeconomic environment, country-level data were obtained from the World Bank World Development Indicators.

Dependent variables

At the population level, mortality rates described earlier were obtained from UNICEF (UNICEF, 1994). As previously mentioned, the primary outcome investigated was perceived health status, specifically perceived overall health in the previous 12 months. Perceived health was rated on a five-point scale: very poor, poor, average, good and very good. The perceived health variable was then dichotomised with those reporting very poor or poor health classified as having 'poor health' and all other responses combined.

Lifecourse variable

Education was conceptualised as a developmental variable, instead of an aspect of current socioeconomic status, because it represents the investment in the individual's cognitive development during the first decades of life. Material deprivation, described later, represents current circumstances. Education was classified into four groups: primary, vocational, secondary (A-level equivalent) and university.

Independent variables

Economic circumstances at the individual level were captured using a measure of material deprivation and of perceived coping over one's life. The material deprivation score was calculated by adding responses to questions about how often the participants go without food, heating or necessary clothes/shoes; the score had values from 0 (low) to 9 (high material deprivation). Perceived coping was calculated by summing the responses to six questions asked by the Russia Barometer Survey on this topic. For each question, 0 signified low coping, and 5, high coping. Subjects were classified according to whether or not they earned enough from their regular job and/or portfolio of activities and savings. Those who reported that they did not were defined as 'not coping'. Material deprivation and perceived coping were treated as continuous variables, and classified into quartiles.

Two indicators of individuals' social networks were analysed. Both of these were derived from the Russia Barometer Survey. The first pertained to the extent of reliance on formal institutions. The survey question asked 'on whom do you rely first of all when having problems?'. Subjects were dichotomised into two groups: those who rely on formal institutions only (employer, state, public organisations, charities or church), and others. The hypothesis was that reliance on formal institutions created vulnerability during this time, as these institutions were not functioning well and exclusive reliance on them strongly implied social isolation. Also, marital status, as perhaps the most significant social bond, was used as a measure of social connectedness at the individual level. Marital status was categorised into married and not married.

The middle concentric circle, representing the influence of civil society on population health, was based on measures of trust in 11 key institutions of Russian society. Factor analysis showed two distinct patterns: one reflecting trust for the 'traditional' institutions of Russian society (for example, police, courts, army); the other reflecting trust for the institutions of the 'new' Russia (the President and private entrepreneurs). Accordingly, we constructed a 'view of civil society' variable (known as 'stance') by subtracting the average score for trust in the 'traditional' institutions from the score for trust in the 'new' Russia. Individuals could then be scored in terms of how 'traditional' their views of civil society were.

Two indicators of the broad socioeconomic environment were utilised that have been shown to be significant for health and that showed signs of drastic change during that period of time in CEE: per-capita Gross Domestic Product (GDP) and income inequality. Data for these variables were obtained from the World Bank World Development Indicators. GDP per capita is a measure of national income. Prior studies have indicated that, in countries with lower levels of economic development, additional increases in GDP per capita are associated with improved population health (Wilkinson, 1996). In addition, income inequality at the national level, often measured by the Gini coefficient, is related to health status in countries with high levels of this form of inequality (Rodgers, 1979).

Data analysis

Associations between poor health and the factors reflecting the innermost and middle circles were each analysed using logistic regression. Multivariate analysis was also employed, combining all variables in question. Analyses were stratified by gender, to determine if factors at the individual and civil society levels might produce different effects on the health of women compared to men. Analyses were also age adjusted. As discussed earlier, the effects of the broader socioeconomic environment were assessed in descriptive terms.

Results

In general terms, each of the variables was associated with self-rated health, and the patterns for males and females were broadly similar. However, the effect sizes were somewhat larger for men, especially in relation to material deprivation and sole reliance on formal institutions. For both men and women, the protective effect of marriage was not significant at $p<0.05$.

Multivariate analyses demonstrated that all of the variables helped explain self-rated health. The correlation matrix revealed that no pair of variables correlated more than 0.26, and standard errors and measures of association for all variables (except 'not coping') did not change significantly between the age-adjusted analyses and the full models. The effect sizes for males and females were closer to one another in the multivariate analyses than they were in the univariate analyses, but the trend for larger effect sizes for men compared to women was still present. From this analysis, the determinants of self-rated health appear to have been similar for men and women.

When the two sexes are re-combined to improve statistical power, each of the dimensions originally proposed is represented in the best fit model: lifecourse (represented by education), individual social networks (marriage and reliance on formal institutions), civil society (trust of formal institutions) and individual socioeconomic circumstances (material deprivation and control).

Table 10.1 provides an ecologic understanding of trust in institutions across CEE by comparing several nations in this region to Western Europe. This is by no means a comprehensive indicator of the attributes of civil societies. Yet, there is a striking pattern which demonstrates that, in CEE, the level of distrust in CEE was markedly greater than in Western Europe. The impression created is one of societies where the institutions that individuals need to rely on, in order to cope with daily life, do not function adequately on their behalf.

As aforementioned, a descriptive, cross-national comparative approach was also utilised to understand the associations between national-level factors and individual well-being. From the late 1950s until the mid-1960s, national differences in economic growth among CEE countries were difficult to detect, and their per-capita GDPs were below US$1,000 for each nation. Starting in the mid-1960s, the region began a steady increase in per-capita GDP. The CEE economies, however, were growing at differing rates and so, by the late 1980s, large differences in national wealth were apparent among them. Beginning in 1988, the region collectively experienced an abrupt halt to this more than 20-year pattern of

Table 10.1: Lack of trust in institutions of society, Western Europe versus CEE (%)[1]

	Western Europe	Bulgaria	Czechoslovakia	Slovakia	Hungary	Poland	Romania	Ukraine	Russia
Church/religious organisations	17	53	48	35	36	39	19	37	49
Police	7	68	39	42	32	32	43	67	67
Civil service/servants	14	66	41	44	39	46	50	63	68
Military/army	17	27	33	26	29	19	13	45	32
Parliament/duma	13	81	44	53	57	47	56	73	60
Trades unions	18	–	–	–	–	–	–	–	66
'Old' unions		67	76	69	64	60	66	70	
'New' unions		72	47	51	48	62	59	70	

Note: [1] Western Europe, based on the response 'no confidence at all'. All CEE countries, based on the response 'do not trust'.

Source: Ashford and Timms (1992); Rose (1995b)

growth. The per-capita GDP figures peaked in this year and subsequently declined (with the possible exception of the Czech Republic). By the late 1990s, several CEE countries were making a recovery; with steady increases in the nations' per-capita GDP after 1992.

The period of rapid economic decline occurred over the period 1988–92 for most CEE countries, but for Bulgaria, Russia and Ukraine, economic declines continued into the mid- and late 1990s.

Table 10.2 shows the available Gini coefficients for CEE from the time of political and economic upheaval in 1989 to 1996. Across all countries it is evident that the period of rapid economic contraction was also a time of increasing income inequality. However, the changes were markedly greater in some countries than others. Russia showed the largest relative and absolute increase in income inequality, while Poland showed the most modest increase. Nonetheless, as regards to the broadest level of social aggregation of determinants of health, the trends were negative, both for national income and income inequality.

Discussion

Analyses demonstrate support for the bullseye model in assessing how socioeconomic determinants of health might explain the increase in mortality in CEE during the time of transition. The approach employed of combining individual-level data with ecologic information over historical time also yields insights regarding the manner in which social conditions influenced health.

In earlier studies of this period in CEE, the image that has best described the relationship between the three main levels of social aggregation (in other words, the three concentric circles) has been that of an 'hourglass' (Rose, 1995a). This image suggests a society with an elite top, which controls the available economic political structures; a weak civil society in the middle (to varying degrees, depending on the country), whose capacity to buffer the stresses of daily living is limited; and at the bottom, an overwhelming need for individuals and families

Table 10.2: Gini coefficients for Eastern Europe, 1988 to present

	Russia	Ukraine	Bulgaria	Czech Republic	Slovakia	Hungary	Romania	Poland
1989	0.26	0.25	0.2	0.2	0.18	0.21	0.23	0.25
1990	0.24	–	–	0.2	0.18	–	0.23	0.19
1991	0.25	0.19	–	0.19	0.18	0.29	0.24	0.23
1992	0.27	0.27	0.29	0.19	0.19	0.28	0.25	0.24
1993	–	–	0.3	–	0.2	–	–	–
1994	–	–	–	0.25	0.23	0.32	–	0.35
1995	–	–	–	–	–	0.32	–	0.32
1996	0.46	0.4	0.28	0.26	–	0.35	0.3	0.29

Source: United Nations Development Programme (1996); World Bank (1967–97); UNICEF (1998)

to rely on multiple sources of support, from that provided by the state to that from one's most intimate associations.

Prior to the political changes of 1989, the relationship between the top and the bottom of the hourglass was stable, with a modicum of mutual obligation between the state and the individual. The rise in income inequality during the time of transition indicates that, after 1989, the twin ideologies of individualism and free market created unprecedented prosperity for those at the top of socioeconomic spectrum. Perhaps more significantly, however, these new philosophies allowed those at the highest levels to abandon their responsibilities to those at the bottom, exposing the vulnerability of the common person – who had neither the aid of civil society nor the economic and political clout on which to depend. This is further evidenced by the polarisation of the labour market, with a decrease in the proportion of the population who were economically active at the same time as an increase in wages for those who remained active (Forster and Toth, 1998). According to sample surveys of 10 countries in the region, conducted in the winter of 1993–94, 20–53% of households reported that they could not cope economically, even when resources gleaned from the informal economy were considered (Rose and Haerpfer, 1994; Rose, 1995a).

For the most vulnerable members of society, this left only the intimate realm of family and informal social supports to compensate for a lack of support structures at the higher levels of social aggregation. The variations in country-level mortality support the thesis that, in those parts of CEE that had stronger civic traditions going back over the past several centuries, this tendency was less pronounced than in those places where civic traditions had never been strong. In these latter regions, life became nastier, more brutish and, for some, a great deal shorter than before. There is also supportive evidence from past research that suggests that those who were left to rely on formal social capital only were more likely to rate themselves as having poor health status (Abramson and Inglehart, 1995).

The character of the variations in perceived health status by marital status and age also fits this explanation. Our findings suggest that having a weak social network was detrimental to health. We interpret these results to mean that the combination of an inadequate social network, and reliance on formal civil society (that essentially was not functioning) was bad for health. This is consistent with earlier findings that single people were more vulnerable to declines in health status than married people during the political transition (Hertzman et al, 1996). Interestingly, there were pronounced declines in crude marriage rates in CEE (UNICEF, 1993). Moreover, those in early and middle adulthood, who are dependent on civil society functions to earn a living and support families, may well be more vulnerable in the short run than the very young and the very old, whose well-being depends, to a greater extent, on the intimate realm of the family.

A further question is: how much of the decline in population health during the time of transition can be explained by the effects of (relatively) current circumstances, and how much is due to the long-term effects of early life experiences? Since the rapid mortality increase occurred concurrently with rapidly deteriorating socioeconomic circumstances, it would seem, at first glance, that current circumstances outweigh the influence of early life.

However, one could think of the post-1989 period in terms of a society-wide interplay between increasing levels of unavoidable stress and individuals with markedly different coping skills and responses, which themselves are heavily influenced by early experience (Hertzman and Power, 2003). In this scenario, difficult circumstances will differentially burden the developmentally vulnerable.

In the present investigation, education was used as a measure of development, and showed evidence of a mixed trend in association with perceived health. However, this conflicts with other studies that (using population-level data) demonstrate steepening education gradients in mortality and (using individual-level data) support earlier socioeconomic conditions as determinants of later self-rated health (Murphy et al, 2006). This would suggest that the transition has been relatively kind to the well educated, but brutal for those whose developmental vulnerability expressed itself in the receipt of limited education. Due to the partial corroboration between the present study and past investigations, it is difficult to disentangle the effects of early versus contemporaneous life events.

Conclusion

This study illustrates the effects on population health induced by swift and massive transformation of economic, political and social aspects of society following the transition out of communism in CEE. The dismantling of communist institutions and the rapid rise of market-based institutions brought with it both suddenly diminished national income and a drastic increase in income inequality. These new economic conditions in turn led to deleterious effects on the social fabric of society. Specifically, two (related) social shifts were induced: (1) for the majority of citizens, particularly those at the lower end of the socioeconomic spectrum, their sense of their own 'material' security was severely eroded, and (2) general perceptions of trust in societal institutions weakened considerably. Our analyses suggest that, together, the deterioration in these factors played a major role in the decline of health status in this region.

The principal causes of death in this time period seem to point away from explanations that link this societal atmosphere to health solely through 'material deprivation'. This would be supported, for instance, by illness that could be traced primarily to nutritional deficiencies (for example wasting). Rather, our study suggests that one major way in which changes in macro features of society led to ill-health was through the stress brought on by the rapidly changing conditions. We submit, in other words, that a sense of material and social insecurity led to conditions such as cardiovascular disease through the well-documented physiological sequelae of stressful societal circumstances.

Based on the insights gathered from our analyses, we conclude that the root causes of major shifts in population health lie primarily at the policy level. First, the case of CEE suggests that there are significant health implications of ushering in rapid economic reforms. Although it is difficult to provide a fully articulated counterfactual, our results suggest that reforms of this sort may be better tolerated if they are tempered and unfold slowly. Second, our analyses seem to indicate that, during a time of transition to free market principles, population health is best protected by policies that maintain relative equality in income through the regulation of market institutions and systems of social protection and welfare. These recommendations make certain the marked influence of economic and social policies for population health and reductions in health inequalities.

References

Abramson, P.R. and Inglehart, R. (1995) *Value change in a global perspective*, Ann Arbor, MI: University of Michigan Press.

Ashford, S. and Timms, N. (1992) *What Europe thinks: A study of Western European values*, Vermont, VT: Dartmouth Publishing Company Limited.

Berkman, L.F. and Glass, T. (2000) 'Social integration, social networks, social support, and health' in L.F. Berkman and I. Kawachi (eds) *Social epidemiology*, New York, NY: Oxford University Press.

Bobak, M., Hertzman, C., Skodova, Z. and Marmot, M. (2000) 'Own education, current conditions, parental material circumstances and risk of myocardial infarction in a former communist country', *Journal of Epidemiology and Community Health*, 54(2): 91–6.

Bobak, M., Murphy, M., Rose, R. and Marmot, M. (2007) 'Societal characteristics and health in the former communist countries of Central and Eastern Europe and the former Soviet Union: a multilevel analysis', *Journal of Epidemiology and Community Health*, 61: 990–6.

Brainerd, E. (1997) 'Changes in gender wage differentials in Eastern Europe and the former Soviet Union', Luxembourg Income Study Working Papers, Luxembourg: Differdange.

Dahlgren, G. and Whitehead, M. (1991) *Policies and strategies to promote social equity in health*, Stockholm: Sweden: Institute for Futures Studies.

Forster, M.F. and Toth, I.G. (1998) 'The effects of changing labour markets and social policies on income inequality and poverty', Luxembourg Income Study Work Papers, Luxembourg: Differdange.

Hertzman, C. and Power, C. (2003) 'Health and human development: understandings from life-course research', *Developmental Neuropsychology* 24(2-3): 719-44.

Hertzman, C., Kelly, S. and Bobak, M. (1996) *East–West life expectancy gap in Europe: Environmental and non-environmental determinants*, NATO ASI Series 19(2), London: Kluwer Academic Publishers.

Kawachi, I., Kennedy, B.P., Lochner, K. and Prothrow-Stith, D. (1997) 'Social capital, income inequality, and mortality', *American Journal of Public Health* 87: 1491-8.

Klein, L. and Posner, M. (eds) (2001) *The new Russia: Transition gone awry*, Stanford, NJ: Stanford University Press.

Murphy, M.J., Bobak, M., Nicholson, A., Richard, R. and Marmot, M. (2006) 'The widening gap in mortality by educational level in Russia, 1980-2001', *American Journal of Public Health* 96(7): 1293-9.

Putnam, R.P. (1993) *Making democracy work: Civic traditions in modern Italy*, Princeton, NJ: Princeton University Press.

Rodgers, G.B. (1979) 'Income and inequality as determinants of mortality: a cross-section analysis', *Population Studies* 33: 343-51.

Rose, R. (1995a) 'Russia as an hour-glass society: a constitution without citizens', *East European Constitutional Review* 4: 34-42.

Rose, R. (1995b) *New Russia barometer IV: Survey results*. Studies in Public Policy 250, Glasgow: Centre for the Study of Public Policy, University of Strathclyde.

Rose, R. and Haerpfer, C. (1994) *New democracies barometer III: Learning from what is happening*, Studies in Public Policy 230, Glasgow: Centre for the Study of Public Policy, University of Strathclyde.

Ross, N.A., Wolfson, M.C., Dunn, J.R., Berthelot, J.M., Kaplan, G.A. and Lynch, J.W. (2000) 'Relation between income inequality and mortality in Canada and in the United States: cross sectional assessment using Census data and vital statistics', *British Medical Journal* 320: 898-902.

Sachs, J.D. (2001) *Macroeconomics and health: Investing in health for economic development*, Report of the Commission on Macroeconomics and Health, Geneva: WHO.

Siddiqi, A. and Hertzman, C. (2007) 'Towards an epidemiological understanding of the effects of long-term institutional changes on population health: a case study of Canada versus the USA', *Social Science & Medicine* 64(3): 589–603.

UNICEF (United Nations Children's Fund) (1993) *Central and Eastern Europe in transition: Public policy and social conditions*, Florence: UNICEF International Child Development Centre.

UNICEF (1994) *Central and Eastern Europe in transition: Crisis in mortality, health and nutrition*, Florence: UNICEF International Child Development Centre.

UNICEF (1998) *Education for all?*, Regional Monitoring Project No 5, Florence: UNICEF International Child Development Centre.

United Nations Development Programme (1996) *Human Development Report*, New York, NY: Oxford University Press.

Wilkinson R.G. (1996) *Unhealthy societies: The afflictions of inequality*, London: Routledge.

World Bank (1967-97) *World Development Reports*, New York: Oxford University Press.

Pathway 4
Healthy and unhealthy societies

ELEVEN

The impact of inequality: empirical evidence

Richard Wilkinson

Introduction

Attitudes to inequality are perhaps at the core of the political divide between Left and Right. But what inequality does or does not do to us has remained largely a matter of conjecture and personal opinion. Now, however, that is changing. For the first time, we have comparable measures of the scale of inequality in different societies and can actually see what effect it has. Many people believe that inequality is socially divisive and adds to the problems associated with relative deprivation. New empirical evidence not only confirms that this is true, it also suggests that inequality is the most important explanation of why, despite their material success, some societies seem to be social failures. The effects of inequality on the social fabric are so clear and so strong that the research findings begin to suggest how we might not only transform society and the quality of our lives, but also rein in the consumerism that increasingly threatens the environment.

What greater equality brings

In societies where income differences between rich and poor are smaller, the statistics show not only that social capital is stronger and people are much more likely to trust each other, but also that there is less violence (including substantially lower homicide rates), that health is better, life expectancy is several years longer, prison populations are smaller, birth rates among teenagers are lower, levels of educational attainment among schoolchildren tend to be higher and, lastly, there is more social mobility. In all these fields we find that where income differences are narrower, outcomes are better (Wilkinson, 2005; Wilkinson and Pickett, 2007).

That is a lot to attribute to inequality, but all these relationships show up clearly in the data, they are statistically significant and cannot be dismissed as chance findings. Some have already been shown in large numbers of studies – there are, for instance, over 170 looking at the tendency for health to be better in more equal societies and something like 40 looking at the relation between violence and inequality (Hsieh and Pugh, 1993; Wilkinson and Pickett, 2006). At a minimum, these different social outcomes have been shown to be related to income inequality both among the richest developed countries and, independently, among the 50 states of the US.

As you might expect, inequality makes a larger contribution to some problems than others and is far from being the only factor involved. Inequality seems to explain between a quarter and a half of the differences between societies in average rates of various problems. The relationships tend to be strongest among problems like violence, the health of men of working age and teenage pregnancies, which show the sharpest class differences and are more common at the bottom than the top of the social ladder.

The picture suggests that greater inequality tends to increase most of the problems that show a social gradient and are associated with relative deprivation. The result is that the most unequal societies tend to do worse on most of the outcomes, so countries that have less good health tend also to have higher levels of violence and teenage births, higher rates of obesity, higher prison populations and lower levels of trust, and young people seem to do less well at school. And the social problems whose overall prevalence is most strongly affected by how much inequality a society has seem to be those that show the steepest social gradients within societies.

None of these findings is of course based on comparisons with some purely hypothetical utopian society with perfect equality. Far from it. All the data come from comparisons between existing market democracies and sometimes even from comparisons between different regions or provinces within the same country – such as among the 50 states of the US. What they show is that even small differences in inequality matter. But why? How can inequality be so damaging?

Redistribution, not growth

The first thing to recognise is that we are dealing with the effects of relative rather than absolute deprivation and poverty. Across the richest 25 or 30 countries there is no tendency whatsoever for health to be better among the most affluent than the least affluent of them. The same is also true of levels of violence, teenage pregnancy rates, literacy and mathematics scores among schoolchildren, and even obesity rates. Violence, poor health or school failure are not problems that can be solved by economic growth alone – by everyone getting richer without redistribution. Rich countries have reached a level of development beyond which further rises in absolute living standards do not help reduce social problems nor add to well-being or happiness. This contrasts with the situation in poorer countries where further development still brings real benefits.

Although in rich countries none of these social problems are helped by economic growth and rises in average incomes, *within* each country their incidence remains closely associated with income. Differences in average incomes between rich developed countries do not seem to make a difference, but the scale of income differences among the population within any of them does. The implication is that income matters where it serves as an indicator of social status or position within a society, but not when it tells us – for instance – that Americans have bigger cars and television sets than Europeans. The lower people's social status within a society, the more common these problems become. It looks as if what makes a difference is the scale of social status differences and divisions within a society, and income distribution provides a measure and determinant of the scale of social stratification within each society. So, for example, why the US has the highest homicide rates, the highest teenage pregnancy rates and the highest rates of imprisonment, and comes about 26th in the international league table of life expectancy, is because it also has the biggest income differences. In contrast, countries like Japan, Norway and Sweden, although not as rich as the US, all have smaller income differences and do well on all these measures. Even among the 50 states of the US, those with smaller income differences perform as well as more egalitarian countries on most of these measures. In each case, the countries (or US states) that tend to do well on one of these measures tend to do well on all of them – and vice versa.

If researchers working on the effects of inequality had started with problems that obviously involved behaviour – problems such as violence, teenage pregnancies or the poor educational performance of schoolchildren – the importance of relative income or social position might have seemed more obvious from the start. But for those of us trying to explain health inequalities (the five- or ten-year differences in average life expectancy between social classes) it seemed very likely that they were the direct result of the way differences in material living standards may affect health through such things as poor housing, diet and air pollution. Health was initially regarded as an almost exclusively physical phenomenon requiring physical explanations. That seemed to mean focusing on absolute material living standards rather than on relativities – whether in terms of relative poverty, inequality or social status differentiation. If we had started out looking at essentially behavioural social problems related to deprivation, then the need for psychosocial explanations that could engage with relativities would have been clear. As it is, the influence of inequality on health has only become understandable as we have come to understand more of the physiological effects of psychosocial risk factors involving chronic stress.

In the event, what first aroused suspicion among researchers that the health differences might not be simply a reflection of the direct effects of material circumstances was that health inequalities are not just inequalities between the poor and the rest of society. Instead, the health gradient runs right across society, from the bottom to the top, way beyond those whose material circumstances might be expected to compromise health. A series of studies looking just at office-based civil servants in secure jobs, a population that excluded homeless people, unemployed people and those on social security benefits, found that life expectancy decreases at every step down the social ladder. Even those in the executive grades were found to have substantially poorer health than more senior administrative staff (Marmot, 2004). The material privations of having a house with a smaller lawn to mow, or one less car, hardly seemed plausible explanations for these differences.

Chronic stress

What added weight to doubts about relying on wholly material explanations was when statistical research began to show the importance to health of all sorts of psychological and social factors. Friendship, sense of control and good early childhood experience were all found to be highly protective, while things like hostility, anxiety, depression and major difficulties were damaging. At the same time, biologists were gradually identifying the many pathways through which chronic stress makes us more vulnerable to disease – and not just to one or two diseases (Brunner and Marmot, 2006). The emerging picture showed that stress increases our vulnerability to so many diseases that it has been likened to more rapid ageing.

The evidence of the effects of psychosocial risk factors, working through the biology of chronic stress, raised the possibility that health inequalities reflected not just the effects of the purely physical hazards to which people were exposed, but also the psychological and emotional impact of living in those circumstances.

Very soon this picture received powerful confirmation from studies of non-human primates (Sapolsky, 2004). Although among humans you cannot unambiguously separate out the effects of social status from better material conditions, among animals you can. Studies in which social status among macaque monkeys was experimentally manipulated by moving animals between groups while ensuring material conditions and diets were kept the same, showed that the stress of low social status can produce physiological effects similar to those associated with low status in humans. Since then, studies of other species of non-human primates have shown that the stress effects of social status vary according to the nature of the dominance hierarchy and the quality of social relations (Abbott et al, 2003).

Three components of this picture were then in place. We had evidence that it was relative income within countries that mattered (rather than differences in material living standards between countries); that there were powerful psychosocial risk factors for disease; and, from animal studies, that social status itself – working through stress – could be a major influence on health. Together, these changed the way data which seemed to show that more equal societies were healthier were interpreted. Instead of looking like a statistical oddity, it began to look like a confirmation of what we should perhaps have expected all along.

Social relations and hierarchy

The growing awareness of the importance of the social environment to health raised the question of whether the quality of social relations differed between more, and less, equal societies. The data from a number of different sources left no room for doubt: people in more unequal societies trust each other less, they are less likely to be involved in community life and rates of violence are higher (Wilkinson, 2005). All suggest that inequality damages the quality of social relations. Indeed, this must be one of the most important ways in which inequality affects the quality of life for all of us. Government surveys which ask people whether they agree that 'most people would take advantage of you if they got a chance' show that in the most unequal of the 50 states of the US, 35% or 40% of the population feel they cannot trust other people, compared to perhaps only 10% in the more equal states (Kawachi et al, 1997). The international differences are at least as large (Uslaner, 2002). Measures of social capital and the extent to which people are involved in local community life also confirm the socially corrosive effects of inequality. Given the dysfunctional response to hurricane Katrina in 2005, it is interesting to note that New Orleans is among the most unequal cities in the US.

Some of these patterns are reminiscent of the effects of greater inequalities among monkeys and apes: social relations tend to be more stressful in species that have stronger social hierarchies than they are in more egalitarian species. Among humans, it seems likely that the bigger the income and status differences, the more important social position and competition for status become.

Although not obvious at the beginning of this research, it is now clear that income inequality tells us about how hierarchical societies are and about the scale of class differentiation within them. The limited comparable data on social mobility in different countries shows that more unequal countries have, as you might expect, less social mobility (Blanden et al, 2005; Wilkinson and Pickett, 2007). Rather than being the 'land of opportunity', the US has, going with its large inequalities, unusually low rates of social mobility. Similarly, social mobility has diminished in Britain as income inequalities have risen. And whether as a result of social or market forces, it also looks as if increased income inequality leads to greater residential segregation of rich and poor in both Britain and the US. Bigger differences seem to mean less mixing – both socially and geographically (Lobmayer and Wilkinson, 2002).

With such profound effects on society and health, it would be surprising if inequality did not also exacerbate most of the problems associated with relative deprivation. When we looked at this – using internationally comparable data – we found, as we expected, that greater inequality is associated with higher rates of imprisonment, poorer literacy and mathematics scores, increased obesity, more violence and higher teenage pregnancies rates (Wilkinson and Pickett, 2007).

Inequality and social anxiety

But how does inequality really get to us? Why are we so sensitive to it? Some pointers to the mechanisms involved are provided by the psychosocial risk factors for health. Foremost among these, as we saw earlier, are three intensely social factors – low social status, weak friendship networks and poor quality of early childhood experience – all of which are strongly associated with poor health. Given that we know that these work through chronic stress, the research seems to be telling us that these are the most pervasive sources of chronic stress in affluent societies. Of course, there are other important sources of chronic stress – like unemployment or getting into unmanageable debt – but fortunately a smaller proportion of the population is exposed to them. Low social status, weak social networks and poor early experience are important to public health because they carry large relative risks and a high proportion of the population is exposed to them.

However, thinking more about these three sources of chronic stress, we can perhaps see an important underlying story. There is little doubt that the insecurities we may carry with us from a difficult early childhood can be exacerbated by the insecurities of low social status. To put it simply, neither helps self-confidence or makes you feel valued. Friends come into the picture because they provide positive feedback: they enjoy our company, laugh at our jokes, seek our advice and so on. In contrast, not having friends, feeling excluded and thinking that people avoid sitting next to us, fills most of us with self-doubt: we worry about being unattractive, boring, unintelligent, socially inept and so on.

Perhaps the underlying message from the psychosocial risk factors for poor health is that the most widespread and potent kind of stress in modern societies centres on our anxieties about how others see us, on our self-doubts and social insecurities. As social beings, we continuously monitor how others respond to us, so much so that it is sometimes as if we experience ourselves through each other's eyes. Shame and embarrassment (widely defined to include feeling foolish, stupid, ridiculous, inadequate, defective, incompetent, awkward, exposed, vulnerable, insecure and helpless) have been called *the* social emotions (Scheff, 1990) as they shape our behaviour to meet acceptable standards and spare us from the stomach-tightening we feel when we have made fools of ourselves in front of others.

Confirming this picture are the findings from a review of over 200 experiments in which cortisol, a central stress hormone, was measured among volunteers while they were subjected to various stressors such as loud noises, mathematical problem solving, public speaking and so on (Dickerson and Kemeny, 2004). The aim of the review was to find out what kinds of stressors led most reliably to a rise in cortisol. The authors concluded that we are most sensitive to 'Tasks that included social-evaluative threat (such as threats to self-esteem or social status), in which others could negatively judge performance' (Dickerson and Kemeny, 2004, p 377). They went on to suggest 'Humans are driven to preserve the social self and are vigilant to threats that may jeopardize their social esteem or status' (2004, p 377).

Several of the great sociological thinkers have suggested that this is the gateway through which we are subject to social influence, socialised and our behaviour kept within acceptable norms. The strength of all the feelings related to shame and embarrassment are powerful pressures to conformity (Scheff, 1988, 1990). But as well as the key to how society gets into us to socialise us, it now looks as if it is also how society gets under our skin to affect health.

The development of individualism and the break-up of settled, lifelong communities must have increased our vulnerability to these social evaluation anxieties. Research going through the huge numbers of studies measuring anxiety levels in young people in the period 1952–93, concluded that 'The average American child in 1980 reported more anxiety than child psychiatric patients in the 1950s' (Twenge, 2000, p 1007). Without a stable environment of longstanding relationships we constantly face new evaluative threats from others: we try to put on our best public face and create a good impression.

'Social evaluative threats' are involved in everything from embarrassment and loss of face in a personal context, to issues to do with low social status, as they are ratcheted up by inequality in the wider society. Interestingly, the literature on violence points out how often issues of respect and loss of face are the triggers to violence. The reason why violence is more common where there is more inequality is not only because inequality increases status competition, but also because people deprived of the markers of status (incomes, jobs, houses, cars and so on) are naturally particularly sensitive to how they are seen (Wilkinson, 2004).

Similar processes are involved in the social gradient in children's educational performance. A study for the World Bank showed that when children in rural India were unaware of the caste differences between them, high and low castes performed equally well in solving a series of puzzles. However, when made aware of their different caste backgrounds, the performance of children from low castes was substantially reduced (Hoff and Pandey, 2004).

We can see, then, that increased social hierarchy and inequality substantially raises the stakes and anxieties about personal worth. We all want to feel valued and appreciated, but a society that makes large numbers of people feel that they are looked down on, regarded as inferior, stupid and failures, not only causes suffering and wastage, but also incurs the costs of antisocial reactions to the structures that demean them.

Inequality, consumption and the environment

Finally, inequality makes it harder to limit economic activity to levels that are environmentally sustainable. We have already mentioned that, despite its urgency in poorer countries, there is little evidence that continued economic growth brings any real increases in well-being to the populations of the rich developed countries. As Gross National Income per head rises, we no longer see increases in measures of happiness or economic welfare, and although longevity continues to increase, those increases are unrelated to national rates of economic growth (Layard, 2005).

However, although economic growth brings few real benefits and poses a serious environmental threat, most people want increased wealth more than almost anything else. Given the concern with status, and the use of consumption to express status, much of the desire for higher incomes is of course a desire for the advantages and position enjoyed by the better off in our own societies. Several economists have provided detailed evidence suggesting that status competition is a very important driver behind the desire for ever higher levels of consumption (Frank, 1999, 2007). Indeed, as income differences widened in the US, it looks as if they increased the pressure to consume: aspirational incomes and debt went up, while savings went down (Schor, 1998). Advertisers, endlessly suggesting that products enhance attractiveness, sophistication and exclusivity, are very aware of our social insecurities. They know that we hope – consciously or not – that our purchases will shore up our self-image and social identity.

If what we want is an income that improves our standing and social attractiveness in relation to others, then it is simply not legitimate to treat our individual desires for higher incomes as if together they amount to a societal desire for economic growth.

Consumerism is driven substantially by social neuroses and insecurities fanned by inequality and increased competition for status. Rather than a sign of our rampant materialism, our insatiable capacity to consume is an indication that we use our purchases as a source of comfort – as in 'eating for comfort' – and to provide a sense of well-being that we cannot get from society (hence 'retail therapy'). Our possessions make us feel like more substantial people in each other's eyes. As such, our apparent materialism is actually an expression of what a highly social species we are.

Without a reduction in inequality, the individualism of the market becomes dysfunctional. Status competition increases and social relations deteriorate. If we are to avoid further damage to the natural environment we must first improve the real social quality of our lives so that consumption is no longer used to bolster social identity in a hierarchical context. That means reducing inequality and, with it, the need to resort to consumption as a substitute for the social sources of comfort that inequality has weakened.

References

Abbott, D.H., Keverne, E.B., Bercovitch, F.B., Shively, C.A., Medoza, S.P., Saltzman, W. et al (2003) 'Are subordinates always stressed? A comparative analysis of rank differences in cortisol levels among primates', *Hormones and Behavior* 43: 67-82.

Blanden, J., Gregg, P. and Machin, S. (2005) 'Intergenerational mobility in Europe and North America', Working Paper, London: Centre for Economic Performance, London School of Economics and Political Science.

Brunner, E. and Marmot, M. (2006) 'Social organization, stress, and health', in M.G. Marmot and R.G. Wilkinson (eds) *The social determinants of health* (2nd edition), Oxford: Oxford University Press: 6–30.

Dickerson, S.S. and Kemeny, M.E. (2004) 'Acute stressors and cortisol responses: a theoretical integration and synthesis of laboratory research', *Psychological Bulletin* 130(3): 355-91.

Frank, R.H. (1999) *Luxury fever: Why money fails to satisfy in an era of success*, New York, NY: Free Press.

Frank, R.H. (2007) *Falling behind: How rising inequality harms the middle class*, Berkeley, CA: University of California Press.

Hoff, K. and Pandey, P. (2004) *Belief systems and durable inequalities: An experimental investigation of Indian caste*, World Bank Policy Research Working Paper 3351, Washington, DC: World Bank.

Hsieh, C.C. and Pugh, M.D. (1993) 'Poverty, income inequality, and violent crime: a meta-analysis of recent aggregate data studies', *Criminal Justice Review* 18: 182-202.

Kawachi, I., Kennedy, B.P., Lochner, K. and Prothrow-Stith, D. (1997) 'Social capital, income inequality and mortality', *American Journal of Public Health* 87: 1491-8.

Layard, R. (2005) *Happiness: Lessons from a new science*, London: Allen Lane.

Lobmayer, P. and Wilkinson, R.G. (2002) 'Inequality, residential segregation by income, and mortality in US cities', *Journal of Epidemiology and Community Health* 56(3): 183-7.

Marmot, M.G. (2004) *The status syndrome*, London: Bloomsbury.

Sapolsky, R.M. (2004) *Why zebras don't get ulcers: A guide to stress, stress-related disease and coping* (3rd edition), New York: W.H. Freeman.

Scheff, T.J. (1988) 'Shame and conformity: the deference–emotion system', *American Sociological Review* 53: 395-406.

Scheff, T.J. (1990) *Microsociology: Discourse, emotion and social structure*. Chicago, IL: University of Chicago Press.

Schor, J. (1998) *The overspent American: When buying becomes you*, New York, NY: Basic Books.

Twenge, J.M. (2000) 'The age of anxiety? Birth cohort change in anxiety and neuroticism, 1952-1993', *Journal of Personality and Social Psychology* 79(6): 1007-21.

Uslaner, E. (2002) *The moral foundations of trust*, Cambridge: Cambridge University Press.

Wilkinson, R.G. (2004) 'Why is violence more common where inequality is greater?', *Annals of the New York Academy of Sciences* 1036: 1-12.

Wilkinson, R.G. (2005) *The impact of inequality: How to make sick societies healthier*, London and New York, NY: Routledge and The New Press.

Wilkinson, R.G. and Pickett, K.E. (2006) 'Income Inequality and health: a review and explanation of the evidence', *Social Science and Medicine* 62: 1768-84.

Wilkinson, R.G. and Pickett, K.E. (2007) 'The problems of relative deprivation: why some societies do better than others', *Social Science and Medicine* - special issue, 65: 1965-78.

TWELVE

'Public goods', metropolitan inequality and population health in comparative perspective: policy and theory

James R. Dunn and Nancy A. Ross

Introduction

> There is no such thing as society: there are individual men and women, and there are families. (Margaret Thatcher, 1987, www.margaretthatcher. org/speeches/displaydocument.asp?docid=106689)

Margaret Thatcher's infamous words suggest a declining capacity to conceptualise and articulate notions of the public good in affluent societies. Such a lack of collective imagery is at odds with recent research investigating the relationship between societal income distribution and population health in industrialised countries. This research suggests that societies (national and subnational jurisdictions) with more egalitarian income distributions have better average health status. It is already well established that for individuals in industrialised countries, greater social status (however measured, that is, income, education and so on) is associated with better health status (almost irrespective of health status measure), but at the aggregate level, relative income (income inequality) appears to be more strongly associated with health status than measures of absolute income like median income (for example, Kaplan et al, 1996; Wilkinson, 1996; Lynch et al, 1998). The individual 'social gradient in health' has been virtually ubiquitous across the industrialised countries for most of the last century. In short, for individuals, it is clear that wealthier is typically healthier, while at the population level, it appears that societies with a more egalitarian distribution of income are healthier than those with a more unequal distribution of income.

But the evidence on this relationship is not universal and its meaning for policy is highly contested. Lynch et al (2004) and Wilkinson and Pickett (2006) conducted reviews of the same literature and arrived at very different conclusions about the consistency and the importance of the evidence on this relationship. Both would agree that the implications of the evidence are not self-evident, although they arrived at different conclusions about what those implications are.

We argue that there are three heretofore unacknowledged factors that inhibit any resolution of the debate about the importance of income inequality and health:

- the body of evidence consists of a series of studies that are not directly comparable;
- even if it were directly comparable, it would demonstrate considerable ambiguity in its implications, because the relationship is not universal;
- even if we had perfect information, there are deeply entrenched views about the appropriate policy remedies that would not only be effective but have tolerable side effects.

In this chapter we begin by describing these factors, which, we will show, do little to guide us from the stalemate. In the second part of the chapter, however, we offer a different perspective, which at least broadens the policy options, although they may not overcome the problems created by well-entrenched ideological positions. We do this by examining the implications of a study by Ross et al (2000), which shows that the relationship between income inequality and population health differs significantly between Canada and the US. This is one of the few studies of income inequality and health in the published literature that makes an international comparison with virtually identical data.

While the failure to demonstrate the universality of the income inequality–population health relationship may occur as a disappointment to many who expected greater regularity, it can also be viewed as an opportunity to investigate differences between the two countries that could account for the incongruent patterns. Such an investigation has the potential to offer considerable insight into the pathways and mechanisms that underlie the social production of health. Of course, one of the obvious and fundamental differences between Canada and the US is the relative importance of the public sector in each, as has been illustrated in many of the preceding chapters (see also Goldberg and Mercer, 1986; Mercer and England, 2000). In this chapter we will take as our starting point the difference between Canada and the US in the relationship between income inequality and population health, and will explore some of the possible explanatory pathways that could account for such a difference. In particular, we will argue that the two countries differ substantially in their capacity to produce 'public goods' and that these differences have the capacity to fundamentally shape population health. Moreover, the important differences are rooted in readily identifiable regressive policies and governance structures, which means that their effects could be ameliorated with the appropriate corrective action.

In other words, in this chapter we address the following questions: (1) does the current body of evidence on income inequality and health demand a policy response, and if so, (2) what should that policy response be? In answering the latter, we shall point the debate in a direction that overcomes some of the deep ideological divides about income distribution and policy, towards a discussion of the relative importance of the public and the private spheres in what we call 'the social production of health'.

In the following section we explore the basic dimensions of the problem of what to do about income inequality. In order to provide a possible avenue out of the stalemate that results, we explain the findings of the Canada–US comparative study in more detail, providing the backdrop for a critical reflection on the nature of public goods and the need for a broader conception than currently available. Finally, the substantive portion of the chapter closes with an exploration of the different governance structures and institutional practices that underlie differences between Canadian and US cities in their capacity to produce public goods.

What to do about income inequality?

In a recent paper by Christopher Jencks (2002), he asks whether inequality matters. First, he demonstrates that by nearly every measure possible, inequality in the US is increasing. The same is true for a number of other affluent countries, although the magnitude of change is largest in the US. Is this increase in inequality a good thing for society, a bad thing or is its effect neutral? Your opinion on this, he argues, may depend on (a) whether you think you will know your own position in the distribution and (b) whether you are a conservative or a liberal. Conservatives have long argued that measures such as government transfers of income, centralised bargaining and a high minimum wage, all of which tend to reduce inequality, are undesirable because they reduce 'both the incentive to work and the efficiency with which work is organized' (Jencks, 2002, p 53). Although government policies may reduce inequality, with fewer goods and services to distribute per hour worked, the argument goes, everyone is made worse off. The empirical support for this view is equivocal. The US is the most unequal of the affluent nations and is more efficient than some (for example, Australia, Canada and Britain) and less efficient than others (for example, France and Germany) and there is no obvious correlation between inequality and Gross Domestic Product (GDP) per capita.

On the other point, if you are not politically inclined one way or the other, and if you are not persuaded by empirical arguments, then your disposition towards inequality will depend on whether you think you will know your own place in the distribution. If you think that you will be near the top of the income distribution no matter what the conditions, because you are smart, hardworking or just lucky, then of course you are unlikely to support measures to reduce income inequality, not because of any malevolence, but because it does not affect you. If, however, you think you cannot predict your place in the income distribution, then you may support efforts to target society's least advantaged in the event that you become one of them.

This is a debate that does not go away easily, not the least of which because there are no good empirical data supporting one approach or the other. Another angle on the argument for reducing inequality is because it has an effect on other things we value in society, like educational outcomes, happiness, health, crime and voting. Again, however, the research evidence gives modest support for a relationship between income inequality and all of these things, leaving efforts to act on income inequality vulnerable to critics who say that the evidence does not support interventions on the pattern of income distribution in a society.

For Jencks, ultimately, the question comes down to one of values, and whether, for instance, you assign more weight to improving the lot of society's least advantaged than to improving overall economic output and the average level of well-being. He argues that the question cannot be decided on based on research evidence alone. But where does that leave us? We argue that most of the debate about what to do about income inequality focuses too heavily on too narrow a definition of income, and neglects questions about the overall basket of resources that individuals, especially a society's least advantaged individuals, have. In the following sections we describe some findings of our extended study of the relationship between metropolitan income inequality and population health in Canada and the US. We believe that it brings into relief some possible policy options that avoid some of the sensitivities that seem to be inevitably catalysed when one talks about state intervention to reduce income inequality. We maintain that this is justified and needed, but in addition, it is possible to achieve a number of benefits from a somewhat different approach, which focuses on public goods and what they can do to improve 'the public good'.

Income inequality and population health

Ross et al (2000) compared the relationship between state/provincial-level income inequality and mortality and metropolitan area-level income inequality and mortality in Canada and the US. Previously, Kaplan et al (1996) showed a strong relationship between state-level income inequality (as measured by the median share: the share of total income held by the least well-off half of the population) and Lynch et al (1998) showed an association between income inequality and mortality in 282 US metropolitan areas with a population greater than 50,000. Building on the results of the previous analyses in the US, Ross et al (2000) investigated the relationship between income inequality and mortality for Canadian provinces and metropolitan areas using 1991 data. The comparative study found that at both the metropolitan and the state/provincial level, the Canadian data points extended the overall relationship between income inequality, but that among the Canadian provinces and cities, there was no relationship between income inequality and mortality (see Figure 12.1).

What conclusions can be drawn from this analysis? What differences between the two countries could account for the different patterns observed in each? What further theoretical and empirical questions does it prompt about the social production of health?

Figure 12.1: All-cause mortality in people of working-age (25–64) by proportion of income held by the least well-off half of households, US cities and Canadian cities

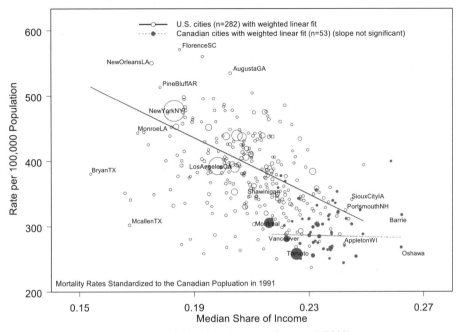

Source: For US cities: Lynch et al (1998); for Canadian cities: Ross et al (2000)

First, as Figure 12.1 shows, Canadian cities are more equal than most of their North American counterparts. This would appear to be a successful outcome of the Canadian tax redistribution system (a progressive tax system and fairly generous unemployment insurance and income assistance benefits). But more than that, this result appears to suggest that income is a much more important determinant of an individual's life chances and therefore their 'health chances' in the US than in Canada (Ross et al, 2000). If we accept that successful conduct of living one's everyday life over the lifecourse in a healthy manner depends on the consumption of resources (for example, educational, healthcare, recreational and infrastructural resources), then one of the clear differences between Canada and the US that could affect the income inequality–mortality phenomenon is that many of these resources are simply available to Canadians universally at no cost to the individual, while in the US these resources must be purchased with one's 'disposable' income. With fewer public goods in the US than Canada, disposable income becomes a much more important determinant of life chances. Conversely, this also implies that there is an important and consequential redistributive impact of non-cash benefits such as public education and healthcare benefits. A good example of the redistributive impact of Canadian healthcare is shown by Mustard et al (1998). Figure 12.2 shows the results of their analysis, which demonstrates the horizontal equity within the Canadian healthcare system: individuals in each of 10 income groups pay into the healthcare system according to their ability to pay, not their use. It is likely that a similar phenomenon would be seen for vertical equity – those paying at a given point in time are not those using the most services.

But how can we conceive of a benefit, if any, that might accrue to those paying for but not using services at any given time (be they healthcare, education, recreation and so on), beyond that provided by the notions of vertical and horizontal equity? The best answer commonly available from economic thought comes from the notion of 'public goods'. A 'pure' public good is defined by three criteria. The first of these criteria is that of *joint supply* or *non-rivalness*, which means that once a good is supplied to one person, it can also be supplied to all other persons at no extra cost – a corollary to this is that one person's consumption of the good does not affect consumption of the good by others. A park is a good that exhibits the characteristic of non-rivalness in consumption, as the use of a park by one person does not prevent its use by another (to a point) (Bird and Slack, 1993). The second criterion defining a public good is *non-excludability*, whereby having provided the good to one person it is impossible to exclude any

Figure 12.2: Incidence of taxation and incidence of healthcare benefits, by economic family income decile, Manitoba, 1994

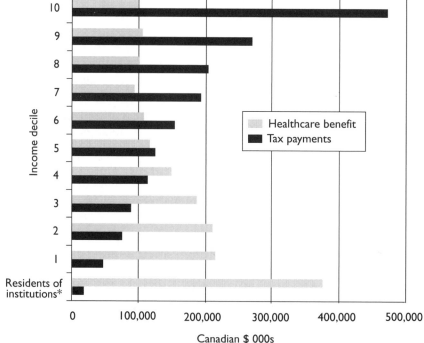

Note: *For example, long-term care facilities

Source: Mustard et al (1998)

person from enjoying its benefits regardless of their willingness to pay for it (that is, through taxes). A person cannot easily be prevented from using a public road, for example. Finally, there is the criterion of *non-rejectability*, which means that once a good is supplied it must be consumed equally by all (Pinch, 1985). Neither a park nor a road satisfies this criteria (mainly because of their geographically specific character), but other goods like national defence, monetary systems, clean air and information do.

The economic theory of public goods says little about whether a good should be provided by the public or private sector. It focuses instead on the characteristics of goods and services that make them vulnerable to market failure and which make it difficult to apply the principles of Pareto optimality (Loehr and Sandler, 1978; Pinch, 1985). In other words, it is difficult to assess the value of these goods in terms of whether they make some people better off without making anybody worse off. The 'public good problem' is explained skillfully by Loehr and Sandler (1978, p 16):

> If the individuals who comprise a community express their true preferences for public goods, they can be assigned a tax-share (or price) according to these preferences. In this instance, the public good dilemma disappears and the solution is structurally similar, although different in character to that solution that would prevail in a free market system.

In other words, if individuals express their true preferences for public goods, the goods can be provided commensurate with those preferences and prices charged accordingly (through the tax system). The difficulty, however, Loehr and Sandler (1978, p 16) continue, 'is that community members are aware of the fact that their tax-share is dependent upon their preference revelation' and that 'they will not forego any of the public good benefits once the public good is produced as it is either impossible or prohibitively costly to exclude nonpaying community members from consuming it'. Consequently, individuals will have an incentive to:

> [c]onserve their scarce personal resources and best serve their self-interest by understating their evaluation of the pure public good. Indeed, it is quite possible for members to reveal no preference for the good in anticipation of receiving a 'free ride'. They can enjoy the benefits of public goods provided through the expenditures of others while contributing nothing themselves. (Loehr and Sandler, 1978, p 16)

Where public goods are present and free-riding is prevalent, therefore, argue Loehr and Sandler, collective goods must be financed through some compulsory taxing scheme.

There are numerous examples of goods for which people will tend to understate their desire. A common example is immunisation. People may understate their evaluation of immunisation because they are afforded nearly the same health protection if most of the population they live in is immunised, even if they are not. But of course this is a risky individual strategy, and it is a strategy that is vulnerable to a sort of 'tragedy of the commons' – that some individuals within a system of shared resources act to undermine them in some fashion, by actively destroying the shared resource, like in the case of environmental degradation. But in the case of other public goods, such as public education or publicly funded healthcare, individuals can create a tragedy of the commons by undervaluing the good and threatening to withhold their contribution to the common resource. This is one way of looking at what can be described as Canadians' increasing tolerance of the intrusion of private interests in Canadian healthcare. Interpreted through this lens, it is possible to argue that many individuals have begun to underestimate their evaluation of universal healthcare, threatening to withhold their contribution to the collective resource and purchase services through private means. Certainly, many opinion polls have suggested an increasing tolerance among Canadians for private medicine, arguably undermining confidence in the public system.

But how can an understanding of the limitations of strictly economic notions of public goods enrich our interpretation of the Canadian and US patterns of income inequality and mortality? Are there implications for the role of the public and private provision models in other policy sectors? The answer lies in a critical rewriting of the notion of 'public goods' to 'the public good'.

From 'public goods' to 'the public good'

Daly and Cobb (1989, p 160), in their book *For the common good*, argue that:

> The world that economic theory normally pictures is one in which individuals all seek their own good and are indifferent to the success or failure of other individuals engaged in the same activity. There is no way to conceive of a collective good – only the possibility that there can be improvement for some without costs to others.

Individualistically oriented, market-driven societies, according to their argument, will often have difficulty producing public goods. As described earlier, it is logical that the difference in the pattern of income inequality and mortality in Canadian and US cities can be at least partly attributed to the Canadian tax system's capacity to blunt some of the inequality generated by market-based economic activity. But beyond that, one of the most important differences between Canada and the US is the relative role of the public sphere. Many would argue that the principal difference in terms of income inequality and mortality is in fact the existence of universal public health insurance in Canada. But the largest health benefit of universal health insurance may not be from the direct effects of care received.

The principal benefits may be the role that universal health insurance plays in redistributing effective income and in materially demonstrating and reinforcing national interdependence. Other public services, such as strong, publicly funded elementary and secondary education as well as heavily subsidised post-secondary education, have similar benefits. In both of these examples the recipients of the service benefit from it, but so do those not receiving services at any given time – they benefit from the human capital immanent in an educated populous, from the advantages provided by a healthy populous and ultimately from security in the knowledge that healthcare is available for both minor and serious illnesses, and that serious conditions will not typically cause financial ruin, for example. Those who are not the direct beneficiaries of a public service, in other words, benefit from a collective decision to acknowledge interdependency through institutions like healthcare and education. There is a set of material and representational practices, however fragile and contested they may seem, that support the ongoing existence of institutions for 'the public good' in Canada that are not as strong in the US. (Paradoxically, some would argue that right of centre political forces in the US have been successful in drawing a direct equivalent between complete market penetration of social and economic goods [and the withdrawal of the state] and 'the public good'.)

Now clearly this is an important difference between the US and Canada, as the education and healthcare systems of the former are highly market driven. But in terms of trying to understand the difference in income inequality and mortality in the two countries, especially at the metropolitan level, there may be some less visible, but equally important differences. Specifically, there is a crucial, but frequently unacknowledged difference between the two countries in their capacity to produce public goods at the metropolitan level. Metropolitan areas in US, due to political structures and a variety of other societal forces, suffer from a fundamental incapacity to acknowledge 'the public good' at the metropolitan scale. The outcome of such practices, we argue, is a vast difference between US cities in the texture of everyday life that is not as pronounced in Canada. The health consequences, using the logic of Lynch and Kaplan (1997), follow from these differences in the quality of everyday life.

In short, there are some crucial differences in the patterns, causes and consequences of inequality in US and Canadian cities that could be influential in this case. First, it is well documented that residential segregation by income is more severe in US cities than in Canadian cities, and there is evidence that greater socioeconomic segregation in the largest 33 US metropolitan areas is associated with higher mortality rates, independent of racial segregation (Waitzman and Smith, 1998). Socioeconomic segregation is partly the outcome of the remarkably strong tendency for land markets to act as sociospatial sorting mechanisms, sorting people of similar socioeconomic status into similar parts of the city (Badcock, 1984; Dunn, 2000). Material practices such as zoning policies, and the practices of estate agents, property developers and mortgage lenders contribute to the creation of such patterns. Media and institutional actors also tend to 'represent' different parts of the city in different ways (for example, characterising them as 'good' or 'bad' neighbourhoods, 'the wrong side of the tracks', 'skid row' and so on), something we all have some experience of. While such representations may be relatively accurate reflections of such areas, they are seldom neutral, as they also serve to reinforce and legitimate the material circumstances that exist there, and to powerfully label an area's residents.

Kay Anderson's (1987) study of Vancouver's Chinatown at the turn of the 20th century is an excellent illustration of the reciprocal relationship between material and representational practices in the creation of notions of both place and race. This phenomenon is termed the 'sociospatial dialectic' elsewhere (Soja, 1989; Knox and Pinch, 2000). In short, however, it is probably fair to say that in US metropolitan areas the social inequalities are wider, the extent of segregation by both race and socioeconomic status is greater and the difference between 'good' and 'bad' neighbourhoods is more pronounced than in Canada.

But we would like to focus on the differences in the character of everyday life between 'good' and 'bad' neighbourhoods in the cities of both countries. There are good reasons to believe that such differences are more than just a function of the simple composition of particular neighbourhoods (for example, high spatial concentrations of wealth and affluence) and, for example, the 'norms' of behaviour that exist there as many argue.

Segregation, institutions of urban governance and 'the public good'

The high degree of socioeconomic segregation in the US is layered on top of a highly regressive metropolitan governance and fiscal structure and a set of practices for financing public services that is very different from that of Canada. A high proportion of the funds used to deliver public services is generated from local property taxes and other own-source revenues (local sales taxes, user fees and so on) in the US. The difficulty is that funding public services from the local tax base makes the fiscal capacity of a municipality very vulnerable to who lives there, and subsequently affects the quantity, quality and price of public services that are offered there. In other words, the services a municipality can offer are highly dependent on the wealth of the local tax base. The situation that results is that municipalities with high social need have a low tax base and therefore can provide fewer/poorer services at a higher cost, while municipalities with lower social needs are those with a wealthy tax base and can therefore provide more, higher-quality services at a lower cost. Additionally, the failure to provide public services occurs at a much lower social cost than in lower socioeconomic municipalities, because individuals in higher socioeconomic municipalities are able to purchase 'goods' privately. The situation is further exacerbated by the inherent incentive for municipal fragmentation and economic flight that occurs under such circumstances, both strategies available for relatively wealthier people to get better services at a lower cost. Ultimately, this situation creates a considerable patchwork of inequitable services and public goods across the urban landscape, and, we would argue, constitutes a fundamental crisis of collective production.

The structure of fiscal governance for Canadian cities is significantly different from that in the US and it may be that this is reflected in the Canada–US income inequality/mortality findings. Although cities in Canada and the US hold similar constitutional status, that is, only having powers deemed to them by the province (or the state in the case of the US), public goods produced and consumed in Canadian cities tend to be financed from the local tax base to a far smaller degree than in the US. Moreover, and equally important, Canadian municipalities have traditionally not shouldered much responsibility for financing redistributive social programmes; they have received transfer payments for such expenses (usually because the programmes are established by the provinces and delivered by municipalities). Canadian municipal policy tends to embody the basic public finance principle that redistributive social programmes should be funded from tax 'instruments that are broadly based and that reflect ability to pay ... the property tax (the primary source of municipal revenue) is a wholly inappropriate base from which to finance these services' (Hobson and St Hilaire, 1997, p v).

Although the governance structure for funding and delivering services in Canadian metropolitan areas is different from that of the US, Canada is beginning to demonstrate some disconcerting trends. Despite a strong tradition of provincial transfer payments to municipalities creating a stable revenue stream divorced from the local tax base, between 1975 and 1994 municipalities in most provinces witnessed an increase in the regressivity of their municipal tax regimes. In a survey of six provinces, Graham et al (1998) showed that most provinces experienced a decline in the share of their revenues represented by transfer payments (the largest drop was in Ontario, from 50% in 1975 to 39% in 1994, while transfers became more important in British Columbia, from 37% in 1975 to 55% in 1994) and an increase in the importance of user fees (across all provinces) (Table 12.1). Changes in the proportion of municipal revenue coming from the local property tax base were mixed, according to the same survey. In Quebec and Ontario, Canada's two most populous provinces, property taxes became a more important source of municipal revenue, while in Nova Scotia, Manitoba, British Columbia and Alberta they have declined in importance. While it is difficult to verify quantitatively, in principle, the fiscal centrality in the Canadian system of public goods production allows for a more equitable distribution of resources across society and space, and reduces incentives and opportunities for economic flight, fragmentation and individuals' withdrawal of their tax resources from the greater metropolitan pool of resources.

(It is considerably more difficult to evaluate the relative equity of various fiscal arrangements than this data permits. To use an example, if the logic of metropolitan fiscal equity were as simple as we have presented it here, then the 'mega-city' movement in Ontario [metropolitan consolidation] would look like an unquestionably good idea. Unfortunately, however, metropolitan consolidation has been packaged with considerable downloading of services, such as welfare

Table 12.1: Percentage distribution of revenue by source: 1975, 1985 and 1994

Revenue source	Nova Scotia	Quebec	Ontario	Manitoba	Alberta	British Columbia
Total own-revenue (%)						
1975	39	45	49	56	45	62
1985	36	45	57	49	50	57
1994	41	53	60	51	50	44
Own-source revenues (%)						
Property tax						
1975	31	32	38	42	29	49
1985	23	33	41	32	26	37
1994	27	39	45	35	24	23
Fees/sales						
1975	5	8	6	6	12	10
1985	8	8	12	10	15	14
1994	9	10	11	10	17	15
Transfers						
1975	59	55	50	43	54	37
1985	62	54	41	49	49	41
1994	58	46	39	48	49	55

Source: Data from Graham et al (1998).

and public housing. Coupled with the erosion of provincial transfer payments, the downloading of services will provide disincentives for a given municipality to offer any service that attracts poor people, such as public housing. It follows that fiscal consolidation may be a necessary, but not sufficient condition for the production of public goods in a metropolitan area.)

More generally, the Canadian system of public finance allows senior governments the opportunity to sort out many fiscal equity issues, although Table 12.1 provides some evidence that this may be eroding over time and we may be moving towards a more American-style metropolitan fiscal regime.

One possible hypothesis that arises from this is that metropolitan income inequality translates into (1) inequalities in the availability of 'public goods' (as reflected by public services such as municipal infrastructure, schools, recreation, public transportation and so on), and possibly, (2) a fundamental incapacity to produce public goods at all. Arguably, this occurs more so in the US than in

Canada because of the nature of municipal governance structures and the way that public services are financed, as described above. In terms of health effects, the inequality or non-existence of public goods would contribute to the overall demand/resource equation for individuals in a way that would increase their demands and decrease their resources (to use Kaplan's, 1996, terms), translating into health inequalities through stress mechanisms. One difficulty that remains with the income inequality and mortality analysis is that it is not clear how inequality affects wealthier people, or, more specifically, whether it does and to what extent. But in short, while the precise mechanisms linking everyday living circumstances and health remain unclear, it is clear that wide metropolitan income disparities, coupled with forces internal to the operation of land markets and zoning policies, can produce substantial socioeconomic segregation in both Canadian and US metropolitan areas. But in the US, a more substantial sociospatial inequality is layered on top of a highly regressive system of metropolitan public finance, producing vast differences in the quality of everyday life across the landscape, and fundamentally undermining any material or representational notion of 'the public good'.

The social production of health and the role of the public sphere

At the beginning of this chapter, we implied that it may be a weakening of our collective commitment to an equitable distribution of public goods and the capacity to live in good health that is the root cause of the atrophy of the public sphere and an emerging 'crisis of collective production' (this is similar to the argument that Coburn, 2000, makes). We have presented evidence that suggests that redistributive social policy, both to individuals and in terms of collective production, may be good for health, and that is why we see the difference in the relationship between income inequality and mortality in Canadian and US cities. But the subtext of this argument is that 'representational' aspects of collective goods drive the 'material' ones – that our feelings of shared purpose and fate unilaterally shape our material commitment to the collective production of public goods. But what if it also worked in the opposite direction? What if our material interdependency, whether actively created or apparently natural, shaped our feelings of collective purpose and our commitment to some notion of 'the public good'? Said differently, such a proposition would mean that recognition of social interdependency is the *outcome* of material interdependency (that is, through public systems such as healthcare and education systems, or at a more local level through parks and recreation services). Indeed, it is a common observation that much of what makes the disparate peoples of Canada unified is their common link to the healthcare system and the 'social safety net' more generally. The strong fiscal unity at the provincial and federal levels, we would argue, provides a material and representational basis for a wider (spatially) sense of 'the public good' in society – the means and the societal legitimacy to produce collective goods. It follows, then, that policy could lead politics and renewed investment in collective production mechanisms could spark a virtuous circle – more public investment leading to a greater sense of social solidarity, leading to a stronger commitment to public investment and so on. The evidence presented in the foregoing suggests that the existence of strong mechanisms for producing public goods would also produce health. It remains to be seen whether such a scenario will play itself out.

References

Anderson, K. J. (1987) 'The idea of Chinatown: The power of place and institutional practice in the making of a racial category', *Annals of the Association of American Geographers* 77(4): 580-98.

Badcock, B. (1984) *Unfairly structured cities*, London: Blackwell.

Bird, R.M. and Slack, N.E. (1993) *Urban public finance in Canada* (2nd edition), Toronto: Wiley.

Coburn, D. (2000) 'Income inequality, social cohesion and the health status of populations: the role of neo-liberalism', *Social Science and Medicine* 51: 135-46.

Daly, H.E. and Cobb, J.B., Jr (1989) *For the common good*, Boston, MA: Beacon Press.

Dunn, J.R. (2000) 'Housing and health inequalities: review and prospects for research', *Housing Studies* 15: 341–66.

Goldberg, M. and Mercer, J. (1986) *The myth of the North American city*, Vancouver: University of British Columbia Press.

Graham, K., Phillips, S. and Maslove, A. (1998) *Urban governance in Canada*, Toronto: Harcourt Brace.

Hobson, P. and St Hilaire, F. (eds) (1997) *Urban governance and finance: A question of who does what*, Montreal: Renouf Books.

Jencks, C. (2002) 'Does inequality matter?', *Daedalus* 131(1):49-65.

Kaplan, G.A. (1996) 'People and places: Contrasting perspectives on the association between social class and health', *International Journal of Health Services* 26(3): 507-19.

Kaplan, G.A., Pamuk, E.R., Lynch, J.W., Cohen, R.D. and Balfour, J.L. (1996) 'Inequality in income and mortality in the United States: analysis of mortality and potential pathways', *British Medical Journal* 312: 999-1003.

Knox, P.L. and Pinch, S. (2000) *Urban social geography: An introduction*, New York, NY: Prentice Hall.

Loehr, W. and Sandler, T. (1978) *Public goods and public policy*, Beverly Hills, CA: Sage Publications.

Lynch, J. and Kaplan, G. (1997) 'Understanding how inequality in the distribution of income affects health', *Journal of Health Psychology* 2(3): 297-314.

Lynch, J.W., Kaplan, G.A., Pamuk, E.R., Cohen, R.D., Heck, K.E., Balfour, J.L. and Yen, I.H (1998) 'Income inequality and mortality in metropolitan areas of the United States', *American Journal of Public Health* 88(7): 1074-80.

Lynch, J.W., Davey Smith, G., Harper, S., Hillemeier, M., Ross, N.A., Kaplan, G.A. and Wolfson, M.C. (2004) 'Is income inequality a determinant of population health? Part 1: a systematic review', *Milbank Quarterly* 82(1): 5-99.

Mercer, J. and England, K. (2000) 'Canadian cities in continental context', in T. Bunting and P. Filion (eds) *Canadian cities in transition* (2nd edn) Toronto: Oxford University Press: 55-75.

Mustard, C., Barer, M.L., Evans, R.G., Horne, J., Mayer, T. and Derksen, S. (1998) 'Paying taxes and using health care services: the distributional consequences of tax financed universal health insurance in a Canadian province', Paper presented to the Conference on the State of Living Standards and the Quality of Life in Canada, Ottawa, 30-31 October, cited with permission.

Pinch, S. (1985) *Cities and services: The geography of collective consumption*, London: Routledge and Kegan Paul.

Ross, N.A., Wolfson, M.W., Dunn, J.R., Berthelot, J.-M., Kaplan, G. and Lynch, J.W. (2000) 'Relation between income inequality and mortality in Canada and in the United States: a cross sectional assessment using Census data and vital statistics', *British Medical Journal* 320(7239): 898-902.

Soja, E. (1989) *Postmodern geographies: The reassertion of space in critical social theory*, London: Verso.

Waitzman, N.J. and Smith, K.R. (1998) 'Separate but lethal: the effects of economic segregation on mortality in metropolitan America', *Milbank Memorial Fund Quarterly* 76: 341-73.

Wilkinson, R.G. (1996) *Unhealthy societies: The afflictions of inequality*, London: Routledge.

Wilkinson, R.G. and Pickett, K.E. (2006) 'Income inequality and population health: a review and explanation of the evidence', *Social Science & Medicine* 62: 1768-84.

THIRTEEN

Inequality and health: models for moving from science to policy

Salvatore J. Babones

Introduction

More equal societies exhibit longer life expectancy than less equal societies. This implies that societies could potentially become healthier through reductions in inequality, but the micro-level mechanisms through which this could be accomplished are not obvious. Nonetheless, it is clear that there exists some sort of relationship between inequality and health, and that it is both scientifically and politically important. Given this, what is the best way to move towards policy implications? Getting from health science to health policy requires first that the statistical model connecting income inequality to population health be translated into a conceptual model that traces out the transmission mechanism through which societal inequality is ultimately reflected in individual health.

It is argued later in this chapter that inequality affects health mainly through its relationship to the character of the workplace, and that the character of the workplace must change in order both to reduce inequality and to promote population health. A long tradition of research on social structure and personality has taught us that (external) work conditions affect the worker's (inner) self (Kohn and Schooler, 1982); parallel research on worker autonomy has more recently shown how such conditions are correlated with health outcomes (Marriot and Davey Smith, 1997). It is reasonable to surmise that working conditions thus affect health through their effects on the self; this suggests that the appropriate location for policy intervention is the workplace.

That said, specific pathways through which such mechanisms operate must be identified and corresponding public policy options must be formulated that intervene at the level of the individual's lived reality. Moreover, and too often overlooked in policy work, ways to engage society in promoting positive change by implementing the appropriate policies must be identified. This chapter offers a framework within which each of these required steps might be accomplished. The ultimate goal of this framework is improved health, but even if that goal is never realised, the policy mechanisms highlighted below – better workplaces, greater leisure time, more cohesive societies – are certainly worthwhile goals in their own rights. If better societies are defined as better environments in which their citizens can live out their lives, then better health might simply be a pleasant fringe benefit.

Income inequality and population health

Most researchers now agree that there exists a broad ecological correlation between income inequality and population health at the national level. Reviews of the literature on the link between equity and health, whether dismissive (Deaton, 2003), sceptical (Lynch et al, 2004) or enthusiastic (Wilkinson and Pickett, 2006), all agree that more equal societies exhibit better average health outcomes than less equal societies. In fact, the correlation between national income inequality and national average life expectancy is very strong. Figure 13.1 plots the relationship between income inequality (operationalised using the Gini coefficient) and residual life expectancy (after adjusting for logged national income per capita) for 136 countries using data from 1995 (the year for which data from the largest number of cases are available for analysis). The raw data are taken from Babones (2008). The observed correlation is a relatively strong $r = .350$, which means that, even after controlling for national income per capita, income inequality explains about one eighth of the cross-national variability in life expectancy (variance explained is equal to the correlation squared). The estimated regression line implies that, over the full range of income inequality levels observed in the world today, there is a 10-year swing in expected life expectancy: highly equal countries

Figure 13.1: Income inequality and residual life expectancy (cross-section of 136 countries), 1995

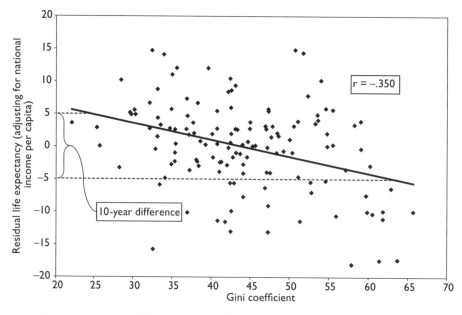

Source: Data from Babones (2008) and the World Bank

have populations that live 10 years longer, on average, than do highly unequal countries. This is an enormous gap, considering that this effect is independent of overall levels of national income per capita.

There is less than a one in a thousand chance ($p<.001$) that a linear statistical relationship as strong as that depicted in Figure 13.1 could arise by chance if there were no underlying relationship between income inequality and life expectancy. This result is all the more remarkable when one considers just how poorly income inequality is measured cross-nationally: there is no international standard method for the measurement of income inequality, and existing statistical compilations are badly inconsistent and incomplete (Babones and Alvarez-Rivadulla, 2007). Error in the independent variable tends to attenuate the strength of the estimated relationship between the independent and dependent variables. Thus, the relationship plotted in Figure 13.1 is a lower bound for the true relationship between inequality and health, which is certainly strong (although how much stronger cannot be known). Without doubt, societies that are more equitable also tend to have substantially higher life expectancy.

What is in doubt is the correct interpretation of this observed correlation. Do high levels of income inequality in the societies in which people live actually depress life expectancy in those societies, while relative equality in other societies actually lengthens people's lives? If so, is this negative effect of income inequality direct (operating, for example, through universal psychosocial pathways) or indirect (mediated, for example, by material factors such as the availability of healthcare)? Or, for that matter, is the observed correlation between inequality and health not in fact driven by a causal relationship connecting the two variables, resulting instead from the correlation of both income inequality and life expectancy with some other, unobserved variable or variables? Leaving aside for a moment the question of the directness of any effect, establishing causality in the relationship between any two variables requires that three conditions be met:

(1) correlation (the two variables must be correlated);
(2) temporal precedence (the causal variable must precede the caused variable);
(3) non-spuriousness (both variables must not share some other, common cause).

The correlation (1) between inequality and health is clear from Figure 13.1. The temporal precedence (2) of inequality over health seems intuitive, but Figure 13.2 adds some circumstantial empirical evidence in support as well.

Figure 13.2 reports the results of a series of statistical models regressing life expectancy in 1995 on national income (measured using GDP) per capita and income equality (measured using the Gini coefficient of inequality and reversing the sign). The power of inequality to predict life expectancy is strongest for inequality measured 2 to 11 years before life expectancy is measured, then drops off. Income inequality thus prefigures life expectancy to a much greater extent than life expectancy prefigures income inequality. This is despite the fact that life

Figure 13.2: Lag periods for inequality and national income's effects on life expectancy (constant panel of 106 countries), 1995

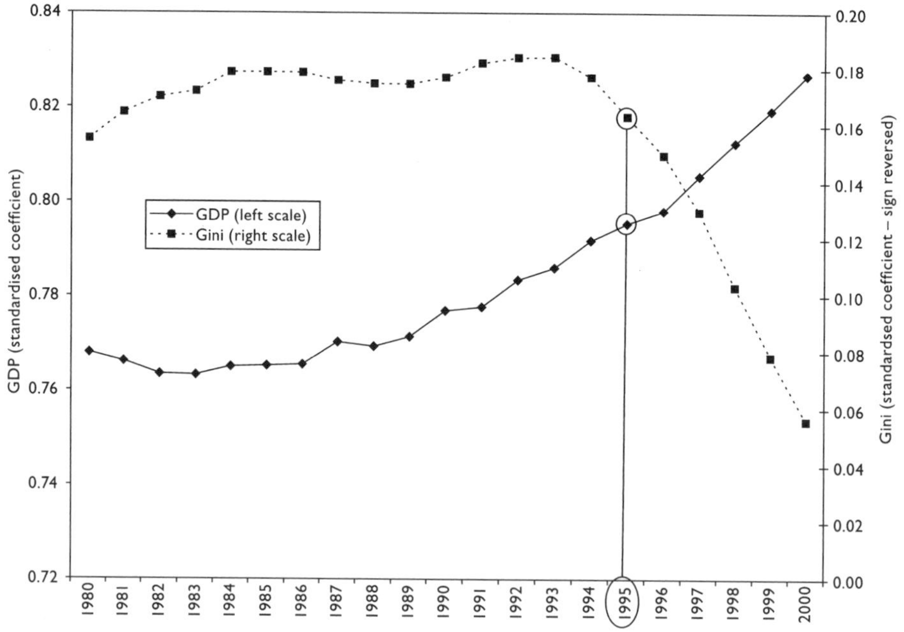

Source: Data from Babones (2008) and the World Bank.

expectancy does, to some extent, seem to prefigure national income per capita. This reduces the likelihood that the precedence of income inequality is some sort of statistical artifact. It seems reasonable to conclude that income inequality temporally precedes life expectancy.

Non-spuriousness (3) is much more difficult to establish. Over a hundred studies (see the reviews cited earlier) have attempted to establish the exact nature of the relationship between inequality and health; it is likely to remain an open question for some time. In addition, a veritable panoply of variables could potentially be common causes of both inequality and health, giving rise to a spurious correlation between the two. Foremost among these are behavioural factors associated with culture (diet, smoking, health-seeking behaviours and so on) and environmental factors associated with social structure (education levels, the availability of healthcare, food safety regulation and so on). Ambiguity about the causal pathways connecting income inequality to individual health clouds the policy landscape: it is not obvious what, if anything, should be done in response to the observed correlation if we cannot be sure what causes it. Any identification of appropriate policy responses, however, must be based on a clear model of the transmission mechanisms connecting inequality and health. Such a model is developed in the next section.

Locating the individual in society

It is easy to make the case that national-level variables such as income inequality might affect individual health outcomes. It is a whole different matter to detect the actual operation of mechanisms through which such effects may occur. With some national-level variables, such as national income per capita, the connection with individual health seems so obvious and so strong as to be beyond reasonable doubt. Rich countries have better health than poor countries because they are richer: their populations are sufficiently fed, clothed and sheltered; they have well-developed public health and healthcare delivery infrastructures; they can afford medicines and other treatments. Nonetheless, formal statistical tests of the effects of national income per capita on individual health still in some cases fail to yield statistically significant results, as in some of the models reported by Beckfield (2004). Such statistical difficulties arise from the mismatch in units of analysis between the cause (national income per capita) and the effect (individual health). The multilevel models typically used to make the connection between national- and individual-level data are of very low power; they require particularly high signal-to-noise (effect-to-error) ratios to detect significant relationships (Babones, 2007). This makes the correspondence between ecological correlations and micro-level mechanisms very difficult to establish.

Where national income per capita is concerned, people generally do not question the micro-level mechanisms postulated to connect the ecological correlation with individual health outcomes, since the postulated mechanisms (material needs fulfilment, better healthcare, availability of medicines) are generally non-controversial, although even here there is some debate – see, for example, Link and Phelan (2002) on arguments over the 'McKeown thesis'. Where inequality is concerned, however, the postulated mechanisms are highly controversial. One reason for this is a basic difference between the character of national income per capita and income inequality as variables. National income is an *aggregate* variable: it represents the sum of a large number of individual incomes. Since it is conceptually decomposable in a straightforward way into a multitude of individual incomes, it can be divided by the population of a country to give national income per capita, a measure of the average level of economic output per person in a country. Since average life expectancy, like national income per capita, is an aggregate variable, it is easy to visualise (and to model) the connection between them: more money means more health, at both the aggregate and the individual levels. The fact that some of the mechanisms through which national income might affect health, such as the strength of public health systems, cannot technically be disaggregated to the individual level (what is a per capita proportion of a public health system?) can be glossed over. The state, acting as the agent of the people, buys public goods on their behalf. The fact that national income per capita – money – can be conceptually disaggregated to the individual level makes its potential micro-level impact easy to grasp.

Income inequality, on the other hand, is not an aggregate variable but an ecological variable: it is an indivisible property of the whole. It makes no sense to speak of 'inequality per capita'. Unlike aggregate variables, ecological variables tend to be difficult to define, operationalise and measure. As properties of the social system, they cannot be conceived or computed as simple sums of individual-level attributes. So to take income inequality as an example, there are at least half a dozen widely used definitions of income inequality that satisfy the generally agreed properties of a good income inequality measure (Babones and Turner, 2003); for each of these different and incompatible operationalisations are used in different countries and even within the same country at different points in time (Babones and Alvarez-Rivadulla, 2007); and even when comparable definitions and operationalisations are used, measurement is highly inconsistent, with measurement error accounting for as much as 5% of total cross-national variability in measured income inequality (Babones, 2008). Given these difficulties, one might think it miraculous that ecological variables such as income inequality have any observed predictive power at all.

It can be difficult to visualise (and to model) the connection between an ecological variable such as income inequality and an aggregate variable such as average life expectancy, because such a connection requires the formulation of a transmission mechanism that connects the two levels. A useful tool for visualising such mechanisms is the social gradient model. In the social gradient model, the expected level of health is hypothesised to rise with a rise in individuals' incomes. The effect of differences in national income per capita on individual health can be represented in the social gradient model as movement up or down the income gradient: countries with high levels of income per capita have more people living at high income levels than do countries with low levels of income per capita. This is an aggregate effect: rich countries compositionally have more absolutely rich people and fewer absolutely poor people than do poor countries.

National income per capita, however, could also have ecological effects on health: as noted already, rich countries are likely have better public health infrastructures than poor countries. Since poor people tend to have worse health, they benefit disproportionately from better public health infrastructures. This can be represented as a change in the slope of the income gradient in health. For example, a breakdown in the public health infrastructure in a poor country might have a disproportionate effect on the health of the poor, since the rich can afford to buy public health services as a private good. The general gradient still exists as before (the rich have better health than the poor), but the slope is now steeper. In practice, it is difficult to disentangle such ecological effects from concomitant aggregate effects, but in positivist, variables-driven research the distinction is irrelevant, since both produce a correlation between national income and life expectancy. As a result, the relationship between national income and health is generally not considered problematic.

The relationship between income inequality and health, however, is primarily ecological, not aggregate, and thus much more problematic. There is, in fact, a highly technical aggregate effect generated by the log-linearity of the relationship between income and health known as the 'income artefact' (Gravelle, 1998), but this has been shown to be small (Babones, 2008) or non-existent (Wolfson et al, 1999), and so will not be treated here. Exactly what kind of mechanism connects ecological income inequality to individual health is unknown. It turns out that it is virtually impossible to connect empirical shifts in the slopes of social gradients cross-nationally to differences in income inequality. The problem is that the income gradient in health can only been plotted quantitatively for a few countries for a few specific operationalisations of health. Nonetheless, the observed ecological correlation between inequality and health implies that at least some people are less healthy in less equal societies. Social epidemiologists working cohort data, most famously the Whitehall studies of British civil servants, have shown that social structure affects health throughout the range of levels in the social stratification hierarchy, even controlling for health behaviours, health knowledge, access to healthcare and so on. This suggests that the impact of inequality on the social gradient in health is likely to occur across the full range of incomes, as depicted in Figure 13.3.

Lived social reality and individual health

The link between equity and health implies that social structures – and not just material resources – are important for health. The link between social structure and health may be direct or indirect: while it is possible to imagine that life

Figure 13.3: Illustration of the global impact model for the relationship between inequality and health

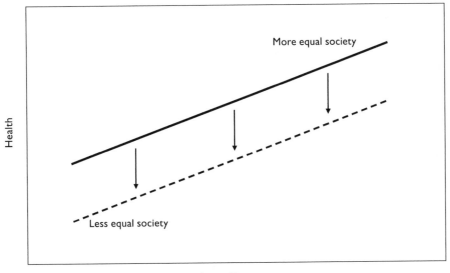

in an equitable society is simply healthier than life in an unequal society (the psychosocial argument made by Wilkinson, 1996), it is also possible that, for example, people in highly equitable societies spend more on healthcare, have better diets or smoke less than people in unequal societies. While such indirect materialist causal paths cannot be definitively ruled out, it is becoming increasingly clear that, as argued by Marmot (2004, 2006) and others, social reality in itself is an important determinant of human health in both rich and poor countries. If it can be shown that an individual's place in society, regardless of material factors, has a direct biological effect on health through such pathways as its effect on the endocrine system, then it is only a small step further to suggest that entire societies may be more stressful, less healthy social environments than other societies. If the character of one's place in a society affects one's health, then the character of one's society surely does as well, since it affects the proximate social environments in which everyone lives. Unfortunately, from this perspective, recent changes in people's social environments, particularly their work environments, are largely moving in the wrong direction.

Since most adults spend most of their lives working, it is reasonable to surmise that the work environment is the main mechanism through which ecological societal factors impact individual health. Recent research by Dorling and Pearce (2007) demonstrates that the relationship between national income inequality and individual mortality rates is strongest in the working years: high inequality is associated with increased mortality among adults aged 20–50 much more than among other ages. This is strong circumstantial evidence that work is the main link between inequality and health, but cohort studies like Whitehall II point in this direction as well. A major finding of the Whitehall II Study was that low levels of control or autonomy in the workplace are associated with poor health, coronary heart disease (CHD) in particular (Marmot and Davey Smith, 1997). Importantly, this depression in health occurs at all levels of the social stratification hierarchy, from line workers right up through senior management. There is also an important social psychology literature recognising that job conditions affect individuals' personalities, levels of intellectual flexibility and even intelligence (Kohn and Schooler, 1982). This social psychology literature emphasises the positive effects for the individual of self-directedness of workers' activities on the job, which seems to accord well with social epidemiologists' findings of the positive health effects of workplace autonomy.

Workplace autonomy, however, seems to be in shorter supply every year. The rise of neoliberalism in developed countries has brought in its wake an increasing rationalisation of the workplace and of employment relations more generally. Unions, which formed the basis for worker self-organisation and self-directedness in the industrial age, are everywhere on the decline. Governments, especially in the Anglophone countries but across continental Europe as well, now tout the perceived benefits of 'flexible' labour markets in which workers' positions are ever more precarious. Even relatively high-status professionals such as lawyers and medical doctors increasingly work in highly regimented, standardised and monitored environments. It would be incredible if such dramatic changes in the organisation of work did not result in changes in people's psychological, and ultimately physical, health. Of particular importance for this line of argument, Kivimaki et al (2005) report that perceptions of organisational justice strongly and robustly predict CHD. When people have the experience of working in a just organisation, when they feel they are treated fairly and consistently, they are healthier. This effect survives all appropriate statistical controls, even controls for other well-known CHD risk factors. As workplaces come to be increasingly rationalised and depersonalised, the impact on health is likely to be severe.

Inequality is unlikely to be the cause of such workplace rationalisation, and thus rationalisation cannot be argued to be the link between inequality and health. A more likely causal chain is that the rationalisation of work leads to both increased inequality and reduced health. Thus, rapidly rationalising societies would experience increasing inequality as the wealthy, including very senior managers such as corporate chief executives, squeeze greater productivity out of ordinary workers. At the same time, this increasing inequality would be characteristic of societies that exhibited depressed health statistics as a result of increasing rationalisation. Such societies would exhibit a depression in the social gradient in health across all levels of income (except for the super-rich, who are too rare to show up in any case in the statistics) – an ecological effect associated with, if not exactly due to, high inequality. Technically, income inequality is in such a model only spuriously related to population health, but income inequality is too closely tied up in the rationalisation phenomenon that it can be thought of as part of the same syndrome. Neoliberalism, the rationalisation of work, and high income inequality everywhere go hand in hand.

It was long assumed that the prevalence of CHD in developed countries, especially the US, was an unfortunate consequence of affluent lifestyles. This perspective puts the onus of prevention on the individual: the prescription is for individuals to exercise more, eat more healthily and relax. Locating a major cause of CHD in the structure of the workplace, and thus ultimately in the rationale of the economic system that creates such workplaces, shifts at least some of the responsibility for prevention from the individual to society. The US has gone further down the neoliberal path of rationalised labour markets, monitored workplaces and high inequality than any other developed country. Perhaps not coincidentally, despite spending more on healthcare (both in absolute terms and as a proportion of national income) than any other developed country, the US has the worst health outcomes of any of them on almost every indicator. The US is, as Wilkinson (1996) puts it, an 'unhealthy society'. Perversely, it is this unhealthy society that is the economic and social model for the rest of the world.

Inequality, policy and the just society

The cross-national correlation between equity and health suggests that a reduction in income inequality, or an amelioration of the forces that increase income inequality, might improve life expectancy and other health outcomes. The sad fact, however, is that income inequality is not declining in most countries of the world, and is in fact increasing rapidly in some important cases, notably China, the former Soviet bloc and the US. The best evidence is that the world is moving towards a US-style social model. As shown in Figure 13.4, inequality is generally rising throughout the world. The regression line displayed on the chart shows the expected rate of inequality change for any given initial level of inequality. Although the data (based on Babones and Alvarez-Rivadulla, 2007) are now quite old, they show that the trend in the early phase of the global rise of neoliberalism was for all countries to move towards the US level of income inequality. For a few high-inequality countries, this represents a decline in inequality, but for the vast majority of countries, it represents an increase. More worrying still, US income inequality has risen steadily since 1990. The danger is that given how influential US economic models are in the rest of the world, the US trend will drag other countries' inequality levels up as well.

Some authors, like Coburn (2004), take the position that the spread of social democratic welfare regimes might reduce both income and health inequalities, but despite the hopeful prognoses of dreamers like Boswell and Chase-Dunn

Figure 13.4: National inequality change, 1975–90, plotted against initial inequality levels (38 countries for which the minimum time series data are available)

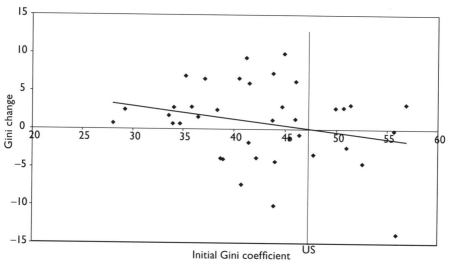

Source: Data from Babones and Alvarez-Rivadulla (2007)

(2000), there is no sign of such a development. If anything, it seems that the opposite is occurring: global policy makers seem to accept the creed of economic rationalisation uncritically, with perhaps some sadness over the fate of new economy 'losers' but little action in terms of concrete, funded policies to mitigate the negative effects of economic rationalisation. The two great forces of global economic rationalisation have been the boom in long-distance trade and the information technology (IT) revolution. Cheap trans-oceanic container shipping has made it possible to locate manufacturing wherever in the world costs are lowest, which, in today's economy, mainly means China and South East Asia. Similarly, low-cost, high-capacity communications and computing have made it possible to locate many service industries anywhere in the world, with the transfer of call centres and IT support operations to India the archetypical example. The magnitude of these international developments notwithstanding, the effect of transportation and IT on the workplace within countries has perhaps been even greater.

Changing the character of a society in a way that improves health, however, may be more a complicated matter than simply redistributing income. If income inequality is just an indicator of a broader syndrome of the 'unhealthy society', then reducing inequality might not have much if any effect on population health after all. Reforming society root and branch is a difficult proposition. More promising, though, are the prospects for changing the workplace, the most likely source of the relationship between inequality and health. From this standpoint, changes in the workplace in recent years have mainly been in the wrong direction. The rise of IT, once predicted to liberate workers from the ball and chain of cubicle and desk as droves of workers abandoned the office to work from idyllic hammocks by the beach, seems more likely to reduce personal autonomy as it dramatically increases the ability of management to measure and control workers' activities on a second-by-second basis. Worse, when workers do escape to those hammocks by the beach, they now often have their work laptops next to them. It is possible that the only workers who will experience increased autonomy in the workplace of the future are those who already experience the most autonomy today: senior executives and top-level professionals.

How, then, can the benefits of life in more equitable societies be extended to ordinary workers who have the misfortune to live in less equitable societies? One way would be through the incremental improvement of the largely corporatist structures in which most people in the industrialised world are employed – and in which most people in the industrialising world will be employed. Unfortunately, despite Pollyanna-ish management theorising to the contrary, greater workplace autonomy for the masses seems less likely as a vision of the future than *1984*-style corporatist totalitarianism. Perhaps greater workplace autonomy will come about through wholesale societal change: the move from capitalist to socialist organisation of the workplace forecast by Boswell and Chase-Dunn (2000) and others. While waiting for Godot, though, we might want to take more modest, more practical steps to improve health. Moreover, such steps need not be pursued mainly for their potential (and arguably tenuous) health-promoting effects. Instead, policies that promote greater equity are seemingly very attractive in their own right.

The obvious direct policy response to research showing that highly rationalised workplaces can be harmful to workers' health is to de-rationalise the workplace or, failing that, to reduce the relative importance of the workplace in people's lives. If the former is unlikely to be accomplished without jettisoning the entire capitalist system, the latter is eminently within reach. Mainstays of progressive social policy such as family leave laws, more generous unemployment compensation, effective job retraining programmes and working-hour limitations all serve this purpose. Moreover, all of these policies are generally popular with workers, and workers make up the vast majority of the electorate in representative democracies. While global social democracy and world socialism are probably doomed to remain permanently in the future, policies to reduce the relative importance of the workplace in people's lives are here now. They are part of the existing policy dialogue. Adding improved population health to the myriad reasons why such policies are socially desirable can only improve their chances of being implemented where they have not been already.

Ultimately, any systematic response will have to be based on changing the regulatory environment in which employers operate. The best antidote to the loss of control of one's working conditions might be a gain in control over the terms under which one works at all. In democratic societies, this should not be difficult. Nonetheless, it is apparently very difficult. Marx claimed that the ruling ideas were everywhere the ideas of the ruling class, and Gramsci demonstrated how such ruling ideas come to be accepted by the population as a whole, even when they conflict violently with the personal interests of the majority of the population. Nonetheless, policy proposals that transparently promote the self-interests of the electorate, like France's law on the 35-hour working week of 2000, will always stand a chance of being implemented. If they have academic legitimacy as well, that certainly cannot hurt. Towards that end, and for the record, let me conclude by stating unequivocally that perhaps the most important thing that democratic electorates could do to improve their own health is to vote themselves a raise. And a vacation.

References

Babones, S.J. (2007) 'Studying globalization: methodological issues', in G. Ritzer (ed) *The Blackwell companion to globalization*, Oxford: Blackwell Publishers: 144–61.

Babones, S.J. (2008) 'Income inequality and population health: correlation and causality', *Social Science and Medicine* 66: 1614–26.

Babones, S.J. and Alvarez-Rivadulla, M.J. (2007) 'Standardized income inequality data for use in cross-national research', *Sociological Inquiry* 77: 3–22.

Babones, S.J. and Turner, J.H. (2003) 'Global inequality', in G. Ritzer (ed) *Handbook of social problems*, Thousand Oaks, CA: Sage Publications: 101–20.

Beckfield, J. (2004) 'Does income inequality harm health? New cross-national evidence', *Journal of Health and Social Behavior* 45: 231-48.

Boswell, T. and Chase-Dunn, C. (2000) *The spiral of capitalism and socialism: Toward global democracy*, Boulder, CO: Lynne Rienner.

Coburn, D. (2004) 'Beyond the income inequality hypothesis: class, neo-liberalism, and health inequalities', *Social Science and Medicine* 58: 41-56.

Deaton, A. (2003) 'Health, inequality, and economic development', *Journal of Economic Literature* 41: 113-58.

Dorling, D. and Pearce, J. (2007) 'The global impact of income inequality on health by age: an observational study', *British Medical Journal* 335: 873-5.

Gravelle, H. (1998) 'How much of the relation between population mortality and unequal distribution of income is a statistical artefact?', *British Medical Journal* 316: 382-5.

Kivimaki, M., Elovainio, M., Vahtera, J. and Ferrie, J.E. (2003) 'Organisational justice and health of employees: prospective cohort study', *Occupational and Environmental Medicine* 60: 27-34.

Kohn, M. and Schooler, C. (1982) 'Job conditions and personality: a longitudinal assessment of their reciprocal effects', *American Journal of Sociology* 87: 1257-86.

Link, B. and Phelan, J. (2002) 'McKeown and the idea that social conditions are fundamental causes of disease', *American Journal of Public Health* 92: 730-2.

Lynch, J., Davey Smith, G., Harper, S., Hillemeier, M., Ross, N., Kaplan, G.A. and Wolfson, M. (2004) 'Is income inequality a determinant of population health? Part 1. A systematic review', *Milbank Quarterly* 82: 5-99.

Marmot, M.G. (2004) *The status syndrome*, New York, NY: Henry Holt.

Marmot, M.G. (2006) 'Status syndrome: a challenge to medicine', *Journal of the American Medical Association* 295: 1304-07.

Marmot, M.G. and Davey Smith, G. (1997) 'Socio-economic differentials in health: the contribution of the Whitehall Studies', *Journal of Health Psychology* 2: 283-96.

Wilkinson, R.G. (1996) *Unhealthy societies: The afflictions of inequality*, London: Routledge.

Wilkinson, R.G. and Pickett, K.E. (2006) 'Income inequality and population health: a review and explanation of the evidence', *Social Science and Medicine* 62: 1768-84.

Wolfson, M., Kaplan, G., Lynch, J., Ross, N. and Backlund, E. (1999) 'Relation between income inequality and mortality: empirical demonstration', *British Medical Journal* 319: 953-6.

Conclusions
Public understanding of the new public health

FOURTEEN

Promoting public understanding of population health

Stephen Bezruchka

Introduction

This chapter addresses the need to apply the information and perspectives described in this volume to improve health. The basic premise of the book is that individual behaviours are less important for producing health than are structures that underlie inequalities in a society. This concept may be thought of as a scientific revolution or new paradigm in our thinking about health, and as with most paradigm shifts, is resisted by both scientists and the general population. Putting these ideas into action will require promoting a broader public understanding and acceptance of the basic determinants of health. The subject of this chapter provides a framework with which to proceed. Citizens of the US, being less healthy than those in other rich countries, are the target group.

What we know about population health

The concept of a socioeconomic gradient, or differences in various measures of hierarchy in a society, is a property of populations, not of individuals. That hierarchical relationships lead to health disparities may be debated, but there is strong evidence supporting that link (Wilkinson, 1996, 2005). The best ways to conceptualise and measure hierarchy and health are still under study, but current knowledge, if the goal is improving health, is adequate to justify action. In essentially all developed and middle-income countries today, societies with a greater hierarchy tend to be less healthy than those with a smaller gap between social and economic classes. Geoffrey Rose (1992, p 129) concluded his seminal monograph *The strategy of preventive medicine* with: 'The primary determinants of disease are mainly economic and social, and therefore its remedies must also be economic and social. Medicine and politics cannot and should not be kept apart'.

The societal factors that impact a population's health relate to how that population shares its resources, and to how that 'sharing' determines the 'caring' that goes on in that particular society. Where there is less economic disparity, there tends to be less social disparity and more support at many levels that benefit health

(Wilkinson and Pickett, 2006). A wide range of terminology is used to describe these social processes: social justice, equity, trust, social capital or, simply, fairness. However it is described, the effect of the social and economic environment on the health and well-being of persons living in that environment is profound, and not adequately recognised by either the lay public or the healthcare system in the US.

Paradigm shifts in public health

The material in this book describes a kind of scientific revolution as depicted by Thomas Kuhn (1962). Kuhn argued that science does not progress with a steady accumulation of knowledge, but instead undergoes periodic shifts. Such revolutions, or paradigm or worldview shifts, tend to be invisible and strongly resisted by those in the scientific community whose scholarship is threatened. Often in other scientific revolutions, such as the advent of quantum mechanics, one incident or breakthrough brings the phenomenon to public attention. History provides useful examples. The dropping of two atomic bombs by the US on Japan in 1945 presented an astounding visual image that had never been previously observed. The visual impact of those two events required a new understanding of the scope of 'scientific progress' than had existed prior to that point in time. Over the next few decades, the concept of atomic energy began to reach school curricula and popular parlance. Eventually, although few citizens grasped the details of quantum mechanics behind discovery of this form of energy, many understood that vast energy could be released from splitting and fusing atoms.

A similarly earth-shaking event was the launch of the first satellite, Sputnik, and then the first human into space by the Soviet Union. These remarkable accomplishments captured the attention of Americans, who had always portrayed the Soviet society after the Second World War as primitive and underdeveloped compared to their own. The launching of Sputnik invigorated the teaching of science and mathematics in the US in the 1950s and 1960s. Again, although most citizens were not rocket scientists and could not have built or launched a rocket, they understood that the world was entering a revolutionary era of space travel that previously had only been the subject of science fiction.

Medical and surgical care changes in the last half-century are sometimes considered another scientific revolution, with profound impacts that have affected our understanding of what is possible from medical care. Premature infants weighing one pound at birth can live and grow to adulthood; hearts, lungs and livers can be transplanted, and severed limbs reattached. Yet the argument can be made that this scientific revolution has been heavily oversold: dramatic efforts that save individual lives and limbs have yet to improve overall population health. Among the few studies of the impact of healthcare on the health of populations, none can unequivocally demonstrate benefits to whole societies (Jamrozik and Hobbs, 2002). In fact, most of the impacts of healthcare have been relatively minor, despite the popular desire to equate the terms 'health' and 'healthcare'.

Even the sacred cow of universal healthcare has not been demonstrated to improve population health or to decrease health disparities in countries where it has been studied (Roos et al, 2006). Yet population health concepts could have much broader impact on health than technological medical advances, if they were more broadly understood.

There are many reasons for the dearth of attention to population health issues by the medical care system and its academic establishment. Achieving success in academia results from asking narrowly directed questions that can be answered in the confines of a grant funding cycle. The published results generally conclude by asking that more research be done on a similarly narrow topic. That ritual leads to a never-ending cycle of narrow research results and academic promotions that continue until the professor retires. Increasing specialisation within academic departments occurs because 'knowing more about less' commands more respect than attempting to understand broader questions of causality. Issues of advocacy or even disseminating findings beyond scientific meetings are considered outside the values of the ivory tower (Bezruchka, 2008).

Because of the medical emphasis on the epidemiology of specific conditions and individual 'risk factors' for illness, most people in the US think of health as determined by the usual do's and don'ts promoted by the conventional healthcare system: eat right, don't smoke, exercise, just say no, and see your doctor. These precepts are taught at all levels of society, and increasingly throughout the world – and at the individual level they are reasonable admonitions. But scholarship over the last few decades has demonstrated that the context in which these behaviours take place is an important modifier of their effects on health (Lantz et al, 1998). Smoking, for example, in a highly hierarchical society (such as the US) appears to be far more detrimental to the health of smokers than when it takes place in a society with a smaller hierarchical gradient, such as Japan (Bezruchka et al, 2008). Herein lies part of our problem in improving general understanding of the determinants of health. We must recognise that correcting this cognitive simplicity in people's minds, that healthcare and 'healthy' individual behaviours equal health, will lead to profound cognitive dissonance – yet this dissonance will be required if the public is to understand health as a product primarily of socioeconomic forces, and not medical care.

Teaching the ecological or population-level factors that influence health is rarely a part of the educational programme in US schools at any level, kindergarten through university. Neither are these factors typically considered by public health departments in their discussion of policy options, nor in clinical training for medical doctors, nurses, pharmacists or other health practitioners. The American concept of 'public health' is in the main defined by interventions that address the physical environment, such as pure water, sanitation and control of specific disease conditions, as well as access to health services and 'health education' to improve individual behaviours. That the social environment could be a critical element in the production of health is not well understood, not acknowledged or is considered to be outside the purview of public health practice.

Public health research similarly tends to focus on various approaches to improving health services or on risk factors associated with health, in which social and economic variables are typically controlled for but not examined. Academics occasionally document steps that could be taken to turn research findings into policy, but they rarely get to the point of recommending how that might be done in practical terms. There is often also an implicit assumption that policy makers, when presented with research findings, will act benevolently (Earle et al, 2006). Even dramatic or highly significant findings typically are not presented in terms of how they might be used to shape policy, nor about the difficulty of creating understanding of such new ideas. Research findings rarely change dysfunctional social systems (Kingdon, 1995).

What, then, will be needed if we are to achieve the goal of public awareness and public concern about the social and economic determinants of health? Many of us in the health field may have to unlearn many assumptions of the old paradigm, and learn the new. Medical practitioners have had to undergo this process regularly over the years, such as when learning new surgical techniques or medical regimens. The challenge at hand for population health may be more like the process by which the germ theory of disease was accepted – which took perhaps a century. Since we have had at least a century and a half of evidence for the critical importance of social and economic factors on health, the time for a broader acceptance of those concepts may be at hand.

Public dissemination of the new science on health

Dissemination of scientific revolutions or paradigms and their adoption by society runs no predetermined course. Logically, however, one might assume that after a few key leaders in the field are convinced of the key elements of the new paradigm, a subsequent challenge would be to convince influential sectors of the general public of the need to consider these new ideas, and to become convinced of their importance. Part of that process might be to point out a few examples where commonly held assumptions are starkly contradicted by 'the facts' – for example, to point out that the US is less healthy as a nation than nearly all the other rich countries. This kind of simple fact is remarkably little understood, and will often lead to a series of questions as a response. Asking difficult questions in public venues can begin the process. While it would be useful to have this happen in high-profile settings – perhaps by the US President in the annual State of the Union address – smaller public venues are more realistic.

Creating public awareness is the challenging task. From an economic perspective, there is no product to sell, no magic potion, pill, weight-loss machine or life-saving medical procedure. There is no mushroom cloud, or real-time moon-landing show. There is only information that, if presented effectively, will challenge most people's perceptions of reality. To affect deeply held belief systems often takes a generation or two, so it will be important to get population health concepts into the public's eye with exposure at earlier and earlier ages. From this perspective, promoting the population health concept is similar to movements such as women's suffrage or the abolition of slavery. These were based on deeply held beliefs that were promoted from a wide range of social groups and individuals, and are still in fact in the process of completion. Some argue for the need to continue to purge racist ideas throughout the lifespan, and such efforts may be needed for understanding population health.

We as public health researchers and practitioners must take the lead in creating public awareness. To influence opinion we can create one-liners that grab the attention of the listener, and back them up with substantial statements. It is useful to keep a list of quotes and statistics with sources for this purpose, for example 'Do you want health or healthcare?', 'We must organise or die'. Developing the message is a matter of trial and much error. It is important in this process to recognise that even one insignificant factual error can and usually will be used to discredit our main message – so accuracy is paramount.

A major difficulty in promoting ideas that reflect social responsibility in the US is that 'rugged individualism' is in effect our first language. But the language of community deserves attention, and messages must be crafted using America's other language – one based on the traditions of knowing and caring for one another (Wallack, 2003; Wallack and Lawrence, 2005). We need to adapt this language for various audiences, so that what is said to a group of homeless people will be quite different from the messages for a meeting of labour union members. The carefully focused framing of concepts has emerged as a very useful device employed by those who shape public opinion through the commercial media (Lakoff, 2006). Our role is to use similar techniques to present ideas about what makes a population healthy.

Disseminating through public presentations

At a personal level, I first came to see the increased hierarchy–poorer health relationship as being important in the early 1990s, at the same time that I came to recognise the limitations of medical care in producing health. My first attempts to talk about this in public began at conferences of medical doctors in 1995. It took me a few more years of efforts to recognise that doctors had little interest in health, especially from the perspective I was presenting. The concepts had no clinical relevance to them and were rarely discussed in the professional medical setting. I continue to include doctors in talks, conferences, publications and the increasingly rare opportunity to teach medical students about population health, but I also understand that there are major limitations of this approach. Similarly, academic meetings and conferences of public health officials and workers offer important venues for presenting contributed papers, taking part in discussion panels and other formats. Public health workers are, in theory, more open to considering socioeconomic aspects of health than are clinicians. However, I still expect resistance to getting on the programme if my abstract does not address topics congruent with the conventional wisdom of the group.

Many different kinds of organisations outside the medical sphere, such as church groups, parent–teacher associations, service organisations, professional organisations and community councils, present opportunities to speak to the members on some aspect of the population health topic. I have, for example, recently addressed senior citizens groups, a conference on ageing, gatherings of public health officials, Unitarian Church meetings and labour unions. Such small meetings represent wonderful opportunities to craft specific messages in effective ways and to stimulate further discussion. There is no better way to gain competence in presenting ideas of population health than to engage smaller groups where interaction can occur. For example, the PBS (Public Broadcasting Service) series, 'Unnatural Causes: Is Inequality Making Us Sick?' that aired in the US in 2008 provides an opportunity to screen segments for audiences and to facilitate a discussion on the concepts. The website provides a community action toolkit and much useful material (www.unnaturalcauses.org).

A host of community service television programmes with access to various individuals and groups can be used to present new ideas. We can access the many radio programmes in cities that host citizen groups to discuss important issues, often with listener call-ins. Most talk shows present an opportunity to mention key concepts, but the editorial process typically allows for little depth of discussion. Some progressive radio stations also feature interview or talk shows that are open to discussing the topic. Once we develop a suitable framework and focus for presenting population health ideas, it is not difficult to adapt the messages to different topics. Every exposure has the potential for making useful contacts that lead to more opportunities for dissemination.

Community events with public demonstrations or marches can present a ready-made venue, including tables at conferences and meetings where flyers, posters and readings can be made available. Those with artistic skills can craft signs for demonstrations that attract attention to gain broader media exposure. Newspapers and television stations want catchy visuals and radio reporters want actualities (statements from the demonstrators) for their reports. For example, my carrying a placard stating 'WTO is bad for your health' at the 1999 Seattle demonstrations resulted in my getting interviews with the local media.

Once on a programme, with a stationary audience, the standard principles of effective presentations are useful. For many groups, going 'powerpointless' may be best. Face-to-face audience engagement is easier with less visual distraction if we can command attention verbally. Telling stories is often the most effective way to communicate with non-professional audiences – as noted by the Scottish patriot, Andrew Fletcher (1653–1716), 'whoever tells the stories of a nation need not care who makes its laws' (http://www.main.nc.us/cml/new_citizen/summer95. html). An effective story tends to involve individuals, require a hazard, danger or threat, a victim, an attacker, a means of doing harm, a protector and means of protection. The challenge is telling a story that deals with both individuals and populations, linking the two.

Disseminating through the print media

I endeavour to disseminate population health ideas through whatever public media I can access. One simple approach to getting into the print media is by writing letters to the editor in response to health and political issues. Following standard approaches to writing effective letters (keep them short, focused, timely) will increase the likelihood of getting published. Such letters are not major vehicles for supporting paradigm shifts, but occasionally a few readers want to become better informed, and request more information. It is important to develop a concise message in one sentence. What is the problem, what can be done about it? I even practise this technique with telephone solicitors, especially those where the call is 'being recorded for quality assurance purposes', since they are less likely to summarily hang up! Population health is almost entirely a political subject, so there is plenty of scope for those inclined to make use of these channels of dissemination.

One prime challenge to optimal use of the print media is the difficulty of getting articles into newspapers and magazines with significant circulation. Personal contacts may be helpful – I was able to get a one-page story in *Newsweek* as a result of serendipitous conversations with a *Newsweek* editor over dinner at a professional meeting (Bezruchka, 2001). Stories need to be crafted in relation to current events, and a gripping lead is required. A standard approach to enlisting the general reader's sympathy is a human interest story – which is a challenge to adapt to population issues. Most publications have strict word limitations, requiring careful writing that leaves much unsaid. However, success at being published in a major newspaper or magazine may well result in hundreds of responses via email or regular mail, as well as telephone calls and other communications. I believe that it is important for us to respond to as many of these communications as possible, in the interest of cultivating every possible advocate for population health.

Writing popular books has been a traditionally successful approach to challenging the public with new ideas and promoting scientific revolutions. Although several academic and politically focused publishers are now interested in the topic, to date the published books on population health in the US have not been in a format that is likely to be read by the general public from whom, in my estimation, the battering ram for change must come.

Disseminating through the internet

The internet represents the cutting edge of communication, but the extent to which it affects people's deeply held beliefs or understanding is unclear. The opportunities to participate in internet discussions are nearly endless. Newspaper articles and various other internet sites often have a web-commentary section for responses that can be viewed by anyone interested in the topic. Those of us who use this means of communication can spread the population health message. The responses can excoriate or support or constructively engage in a discussion, but we can expect to be strongly criticised for views we present that go beyond individual agency as the chief means of health production. On the other hand, the internet is an accessible mechanism for people who want to be involved to make contact with and learn from like-minded others. We might eventually find this process making substantial inroads in getting our ideas greater exposure. Blogs represent another easily accessible way to craft arguments in written form.

A tremendous variety of other publishing means are available on the web. Podcasting allows voiced material to be disseminated widely, as do hosted discussions on the web with downloadable audio files. Our challenge is creating files that might be suitable for general listening, just like the music that can be downloaded. Many of us belong to listserves and we can use them to highlight news stories with our personal commentary. Using the web for information and constructive engagement may be akin to trying to slake thirst from a firehose – but we ignore it at our peril.

Dissemination through the educational system

The formal educational system, from elementary through university level, represents a largely untapped resource for broadening public understanding of the determinants of health. The opportunity for us to engage in formal teaching is immense. As health professionals of all types we can teach and write for specialty journals and conferences, as well as for institutions of advanced education. Community colleges, universities and the like have few courses dealing with the health of populations but a course title such as Global Health can get us in the door. There are endless opportunities – online education, for example, represents a relatively new one. Recognise that it may take a year or more to set up a teaching opportunity, given the individual contacts and relationships that must be built. Formal teaching allows the unique possibility of crafting course outputs that require students themselves to take responsibility for dissemination. I tend to let the students choose the methods they will use based on the principles described earlier, but give a list of various suggestions and possible venues, such as screening 'Unnatural Causes' in small groups. I continue to be surprised by the innovative and sometimes inspiring activities they carry out and find more interest among non-health career students, who tend to be less resistant to the concepts, than health career students.

Teachers at all levels are important influences on developing minds. Over the long term, promoting middle- and high-school curricula on population health may be the most effective strategy for bringing about a shift in public understanding of the socioeconomic determinants of health.

The need for curricular change

'Health education' in US schools, from elementary through high school, is based on traditional concepts of individual health production. Individual behaviours are the main emphasis, and no attention is given to comparisons of health status for populations. There is certainly no mention of the relative decline of health in the US over the last 40 years. Medical care is usually overemphasised as an important factor producing health.

To ask why our health education system avoids addressing social and economic determinants of health is to invite questioning of the broader purposes of the education system. Carol Bellamy, who was director of the United Nations Children's Fund (UNICEF) for several years, once said: 'The business community needs peace to see economic growth. They need kids to be educated to be consumers and workers' (quoted in the *New York Times*, 3 September 2000). I would suggest that if the purpose of an education is to create consumers and workers, then the system is working. However, if the purpose is to instil an understanding of the world and critical thinking skills, then much needs to be done. We might look elsewhere for guidance: scholars in Australia, for example, a much healthier country than the US, promote the concept of critical health literacy (St Leger, 2001). The three levels of health literacy that they describe involve functional elements such as factual information; interactive aspects that understand the nature of a supportive environment; and the critical element requiring civic engagement to impact social, political and economic forces that impact health. Teaching civic engagement as an element of health education is necessary if we recognise that youth represent the next generation to effect social change. Teaching young people the importance of social action, with accompanying skills, is empowering and increases self-efficacy. This framework would provide a simple yet comprehensive organising principle for a viable school health education curriculum that truly addresses health.

Practical strategies

I often begin a session with students by asking them to describe what they do to keep themselves healthy, and then to try to explain what they think makes people healthy in a larger community. In Seattle, classroom settings often have students from very diverse ethnic and national backgrounds. A wide range of responses from children who are African Americans, Hispanics or recent immigrants from Russia or Ethiopia illustrate the many social realities from which they come, and a sometimes profound understanding of the effects of those settings on their lives. A useful homework assignment is to ask the students to graph the top 25 or so countries in the 'Health Olympics', the ranking of countries by a mortality measure such as life expectancy. Engaged students will continue graphing beyond 25 countries to discover where the US stands. Another effective teaching tool is to present a coloured map of the US by county indicating life expectancy ranges and ask the students to explore possible reasons behind the geographical distribution of health that they see (Murray et al, 1998, 2006). Asking why such large disparities exist in the US prompts looking at basic concepts of population health. I then discuss with them the income distribution–mortality relationship among states.

Homework can include short essay questions, true–false choices and other formats that can lead to discussions about specific issues. Facts that can be brought in may relate to issues such as why the US has the highest child poverty rates of all the rich countries, and 10–20 times the teenage birth rates of other rich countries. We have almost endless opportunity here – in many cases the facts very nearly speak for themselves, when provided to ears that are willing to listen.

By comparing information on health-related outcomes for the US with other countries, we are forced to ask why the observed patterns occur. Why such high teenage birth rates? Or high youth homicide rates? Why so much child poverty? These data naturally lead students to discuss economic and political realities associated with the problems – without any need to explicitly mention partisan political issues.

Another teaching tool I have used, especially during a biennial Olympic year, is reader's theatre in which a 'Health Olympics finish' scenario takes place (Maher, 2006). Students take on country roles, there is a race announcer and scripts are handed out to study the day before. Often focusing on three contestants, Japan, Canada and the US, students race with flag-bearing t-shirts and additional information cards that are flashed to the rest of the class. The US crosses the finish line 4.6 years after the winner in the life expectancy race. This exercise makes use of active participation and entertainment while getting a memorable message across.

Teaching methods that focus on active discussion or other participation and that do not use too many visual materials seem to work best in elementary classrooms. If an audiovisual aid such as a video is used, be sure it is entertaining as well as informative. I like to show a 10-minute video segment of a British documentary, 'The Great Leveller' (part of a Channel 4 *Equinox* series screened in 1996). This fast-paced and cleverly narrated programme effectively presents some of the biology behind the hierarchy–health relationship through human, baboon and macaque monkey studies.

Promoting civic engagement

An important element of our curricular efforts is to help students to grasp the basic concept that political decisions about distributional economic issues are critical factors that affect the health of populations. A number of population health themes have been investigated for school use. A useful wealth distribution exercise is to divide the class into quintiles, and then 'give out' US household wealth as it is actually distributed, using trillion dollar notes. This visible depiction of reality often gets strong reactions from students of all ages – including 'but that's not fair!' – and can lead to civic engagement, the third part of critical health literacy. The links between relative poverty and environmental contamination can be presented in a class setting by dividing students in the class into quartiles or quintiles by wealth and instructing one group, the poorest, that, no matter what happens, they are to keep mute. A symbolic bucket of toxic waste is brought into the classroom and the students have to discuss where it will go among the groups. Although the resulting decision has been quite unpredictable, it always leads to engagement and, I believe, a deeper understanding of relevant issues. A simple homework task is to talk about these ideas with friends, siblings and parents.

I have later found students who attended these classes who become active in the social justice movement – and who report that their classroom experience was what got them involved. Another element of civic engagement is to have students produce graphical materials for display. In a module entitled 'World Health and Art Activism', high school students were able to produce creative and effective posters that addressed issues such as student stress, the wealth gap, world hunger and teenage births. In another class, students drew up models displaying the hierarchy–health relationship. We can script role plays in which students learn to discuss the concepts with strangers and practise with each other or with friends and family.

One of the unexpected developments from presenting new and stimulating information is that parents can contact the classroom teacher if they want to know more about what their student has been learning. Teachers also use the lesson elements provided by guest instructors in future years so there is a stimulus for continuing population health education. After your first teaching experience at the pre-college level you may be 'hooked'. Use class evaluations to finetune future lessons.

Another opportunity that can offer an enrichment experience, particularly for students from more privileged schools, is actual travel to a poor country. We have worked with a school in which the students spend a month in Vietnam at the end of grade 8. Before they go we discuss issues of poverty and social factors at work in the Vietnam setting. Debriefing sessions on return are critical. One student, when asked about the 'big picture' in Vietnam as he saw it, replied: 'We went there and like you said, they were poor, but we also saw they were happy, and it wasn't a drug-induced kind of happiness'. The actual experience of the everyday realities of poor countries can have a transformative experience at any age.

Major global events provide other opportunities for teaching this material. The 10th anniversary of the Beijing women's conference was an appropriate time to discuss gender issues in health production. Discussions about our relations with Cuba highlight the finding that it is as healthy as the US despite economic sanctions placed on it by the US – which stretch over almost 50 years. Russia's rise to house the second largest number of billionaires in the world was coupled with an immense absolute health decline. Sri Lanka has health indicators close to those of the US despite the lack of economic growth and a protracted civil war. An impressive number of world events provide teaching material for health topics.

Teaching population health concepts have now been presented at social studies teacher conferences and to various teacher-training environments. Adoption has been limited because of the lack of sustained curriculum support as well as the lack of mainstream attention paid to our health as a society. We are in the process of doing more curriculum development and dissemination (Just Health Action, www.justhealthaction.org/).

There are few standardised lesson plans for teaching this material available in the US. A sourcebook by World Hunger Year produced by Kids Can Make a Difference presents a variety of lesson plans (Kempf, 2005). One book in the Rethinking Schools series has relevant materials (Gutstein and Peterson, 2005), but none directly related to population health. Similarly, *Teaching economics as if people mattered* by United for a Fair Economy presents other engaging lesson material (Giecek, 2000). There are really novel teaching tools for global health available from www.gapminder.org/

College-level courses

It is remarkable how few college-level courses address the broad determinants of health – we can expect to break new ground by working in this area. Even more revolutionary are classes that require the student to apply the information in a useful way. As a part of the output of both my undergraduate and graduate courses covering population health at the University of Washington and at Seattle University, students carry out a dissemination exercise. I am impressed with the number of students who carry out teaching exercises in middle and high schools. They have gone to minority enrichment programmes, to history classes, to social studies classes, to health education classes, and discovered their own teaching styles. To help students grapple with the ideas, they are required to write a paper criticising these concepts. I am in contact with a few other university teachers in the US attempting to teach this material, largely in anthropology, sociology and social work departments. There is more opportunity for these ideas in countries other than the US (Bezruchka, 2006). The analogous course for physicians – 'social medicine' – is being taught in only a few medical schools in the US (Anderson et al, 2005). To my knowledge, few public health schools address this material, although there has recently been a growing interest in the 'social determinants of health' as an academic topic.

Conclusion: a call to action for public health professionals

We who work in traditional fields of public health in the US need to recognise that while our work may be important, health outcomes in the US suggest the need for a new approach to producing health. It is disgraceful that the wealthiest country in the world has allowed its health status to deteriorate to the present level. The way forward will require us to step out of our narrow academic and personal boundaries. We must build cohesive bridges among disciplines, social and economic classes, and between professionals and our education system.

This chapter suggests that the current scholarship around population health represents a scientific revolution in progress. There is strong resistance to new worldviews, and we in the US are no exception, particularly when it comes to the topic of health. We are faced with relearning what produces health and choosing whether or not to teach what we have chosen to learn. Having healthy grandchildren and great-grandchildren will require concerted efforts by the current generations. There is pioneering work to do in disseminating the concepts of the population health revolution.

References

Anderson, M.R., Smith, L. and Sidel, V.W. (2005) 'What is social medicine?', *Monthly Review* 56(8): 27-34.

Bezruchka, S. (2001) 'Is our society making you sick? America's health lags behind that of more egalitarian nations', *Newsweek*, 26 February: 14.

Bezruchka, S. (2006) 'Epidemiological approaches', in D. Raphael, T. Bryant and M. Rioux (eds) *Staying alive: Critical perspectives on health, illness and health care*, Toronto: Canadian Scholars' Press: 13-33.

Bezruchka, S. (2008) 'Becoming a public scholar to improve the health of the US population', *Antipode* 40(3): 455-62.

Bezruchka, S., Namekata, T. and Sistram, M. (2008) 'Improving economic equality and health: the case of postwar Japan', *American Journal of Public Health* 98(4): 589-94.

Giecek, T. S. (2000.) *Teaching economics as if people mattered: A high school curriculum guide to the new economy.* Boston, MA: United for a Fair Economy.

Gutstein, E. and Peterson, B. (eds) (2005) *Rethinking mathematics: Teaching social justice by the numbers*, Milwaukie, WI: Rethinking Schools Publication.

Earle, A., Heymann, J. and Lavis, J.M. (2006) 'Where do we go from here? Translating research to policy', in J. Heymann, C. Hertzman, M.L. Barer and R.G. Evans (eds) (2006) *Healthier societies: From analysis to action*, New York, NY: Oxford University Press.

Jamrozik, K. and Hobbs M.S.T. (2002) 'Medical care and public health' in R. Detels, J. McEwen, R. Beaglehole and H. Tanaka (eds), *Oxford textbook of public health*, Oxford: Oxford University Press: 215-42.

Kempf, S. (2005) *Finding solutions to hunger: Kids can make a difference*, New York, NY: World Hunger Year.

Kingdon, J.W. (1995) *Agendas, alternatives, and public policies*, New York, NY: Longman.

Kuhn, T.S. (1962) *The structure of scientific revolutions*, Chicago, IL: University of Chicago Press.

Lakoff, G. (2006) *Thinking points: Communicating our American values and vision: a progressive's handbook*, New York, NY: Farrar, Strauss, Giroux.

Lantz, P.M., House, J.S., Lepowski, J.M., Williams, D.R., Mero, R.P. and Chen, J. (1998) 'Socioeconomic factors, health behaviors, and mortality: results from a nationally representative prospective study of US adults', *JAMA*, 279(21): 1703-8.

Maher, J. (2006) *Most dangerous women: Bringing history to life through readers' theater*, Portsmouth, NH: Heinemann.

Murray, C.J.L., Michaud, C.M., McKenna, M.T. and Marks, J.S. (1998) *US patterns of mortality by county and race: 1965–1994*, Cambridge, MA: Burden of Disease Unit, Harvard Center for Population and Development Studies.

Murray, C.J.L., Kulkarni, S.C., Michaud, C., Tomijima, N., Bulzacchelli, M.T., Iandorio, T.J. and Ezzah, M. (2006) 'Eight Americas: investigating mortality disparities across races, counties, and race-counties in the United States', *PLoS Medicine* 3(9): e260.

Roos, N.P., Brownell, M. and Menec, V. (2006) 'Universal medical care and health inequalities: right objectives, insufficient tools', in J. Heymann, C. Hertzman, M.L. Barer and R.G. Evans (eds) *Healthier societies: From analysis to action*, New York, NY: Oxford University Press: 107-31.

Rose, G.A. (1992) *The strategy of preventive medicine*, New York, NY: Oxford University Press.

St Leger, L. (2001) 'Schools, health literacy and public health: possibilities and challenges', *Health Promotion International* 16(2): 197-205.

Wallack, L. (2003) 'The role of mass media: a new direction for public health', in R. Hofrichter (ed) *Health and social justice: Politics, ideology, and inequity in the distribution of disease*, San Francisco, CA: Jossey-Bass: 594-625.

Wallack, L. and Lawrence, R. (2005) 'Talking about public health: developing America's "second language"', *American Journal of Public Health* 95(4): 567-70.

Wilkinson, R.G. (1996) *Unhealthy societies: The afflictions of inequality*, London: Routledge.

Wilkinson, R.G. (2005) *The impact of inequality: How to make sick societies healthier.* New York, NY: New Press.

Wilkinson, R.G. and Pickett, K.E. (2006) 'Income inequality and population health: a review and explanation of the evidence', *Social Science & Medicine* 62(7): 1768-84.

FIFTEEN

Health, inequalities and mobilisation: human rights and the Millennium Development Goals

Paul Nelson

Introduction

Rapid, sustained progress on global health and development would require the mobilisation of governments and the financial resources they command, and of social movements and non-governmental organisations (NGOs), whose ability to mobilise social energy and action is essential to overcoming barriers that exclude many poor and socially marginalised groups from the benefits of global growth. The international aid social system – donor agencies, contractors, NGOs and community-based organisations – is often described as development 'partnerships' capable of concerted cooperation for the common good. But donor governments, NGOs and social movements in the poor countries are often at odds over trade, aid, labour, finance and social spending policies, policies with important implications for health outcomes.

Two contemporary approaches to global development policy – the Millennium Development Goals (MDGs) and human rights-based approaches to development – present an opportunity to learn whether and how these two forms of social energy can be mobilised for poverty reduction. This chapter examines the important differences – theoretical, institutional and political – between the MDGs and the standards, principles and practices of internationally recognised human rights.

The MDGs, launched by 189 governments at the Millennium Summit in 2000, are perhaps the highest-profile example of goal- and needs-based action on global social problems. Three of the eight MDGs refer directly to health status: maternal mortality, infant mortality and 'HIV/AIDS, malaria, and other major diseases'; and other targets, such as access to safe drinking water and to sanitation, have immediate public health implications. Many human rights and development advocates argue that the goals are consistent with and indeed a means of operationalising human rights standards and principles.

Human rights-based approaches to social policy attracted rising interest in the 1990s, in the form of activism on economic, social and cultural (ESC) rights, the human right to health, and 'rights-based approaches' to development assistance. Interest in ESC rights became more concrete as debate focused on issues such as the right of access to essential medicines, and on advocacy and litigation that asserted poor countries' right to manufacture or import generic anti-retrovirals.

This study tests two widely held positions: that the MDGs mirror and complement human rights approaches to social policy; and that global development initiatives can mobilise a united system of states, donors, NGOs and social movements. Human rights related to health and the health-related MDGs are widely seen as complementary: human rights establish broad principles and standards, and MDGs create operational goals, indicators and benchmarks through to 2015. But despite their arrival at the same historical juncture, the MDGs and human rights-based approaches have less in common than appears at first glance.

In this chapter I examine the relationship between health-related goals and human rights from a world society theoretical perspective. Drawing on the framework advanced by Meyer and colleagues (1997), I take the view that global social and health policy initiatives are dynamic interactions among governments, civic and other actors, each of which brings specific capacities.

Adopting this world society perspective helps to focus attention on the paradoxical ways that the MDGs and human rights frames for health and social policy have mobilised these sets of actors. Human rights, a system of binding treaties among states, have been embraced and promoted more actively by civic actors such as NGOs and social movements. Softer goals such as the MDGs, which promote voluntary action, have been a preferred vehicle for states, especially some rich-country governments.

The next three sections of this chapter pose three questions regarding human rights and the MDGs. First, how do the two approaches analyse and create a policy frame for addressing current health issues? Second, how do the MDGs and human rights mobilise governmental and intergovernmental action, and social movement and civic action? Third, what concrete policy positions are the MDGs and human rights advocates associated with, on two major social policy issues: water privatisation and the provision of anti-retroviral medicines for HIV/AIDS patients?

Human rights, MDGs and health

Both the MDGs and rights-based approaches seek to reinvigorate the global development enterprise. The MDGs restate poverty-related development challenges in language that avoids reference to rights; rights-based approaches, by contrast, seek to link the development enterprise to the rhetorical power and moral authority of human rights standards.

The MDGs

The MDGs are written and institutionalised to mobilise support from the countries of the Organisation for Economic Co-operation and Development (OECD) and their citizens, by demonstrating the capacity of 'development' to accomplish important tasks. The goals can be traced to the 1995 World Social Summit on Development (WSSD), which enjoys great legitimacy with NGOs and social activists. But the 'Shaping the 21st century' document (Development Assistance Committee, 2006), which became the immediate source of the MDGs, emerged from a process involving little input from aid recipient countries or NGOs. The MDGs, as a result, are widely seen by activists as a product of the OECD governments and the international financial institutions (Bissio, 2003), a perception that affects the goals' ability to mobilise social and political actors.

The MDGs focus heavily on the symptoms of mal-development and underdevelopment: infant mortality rates, HIV infection rates, incidence of malnutrition, and access to water and sanitation. Each of the goals is accompanied by one or more targets, which are to be tracked by a set of measurable indicators. Indicators include outcome measures (such as malaria prevalence and death rates) and measures of direct health services inputs (such as proportion of the population in malaria-risk areas using effective malaria prevention and treatment measures). Two kinds of indicators are conspicuously absent: measures of inequality or distribution (or indicators of discriminatory laws, institutions or practices that may underlie such mal-distribution); and indicators of access to fundamental sources of wealth and security (land, credit and capital).

The MDGs' 'quick wins' strategy, outlined in the 2005 United Nations (UN) report on investing to advance the MDGs, funds 'high potential, short-term impact' initiatives that can yield 'breathtaking results within three or fewer years' and 'start countries on the path to the Goals' (UN Millennium Project, 2005, p 25). These quick-impact measures include mosquito bed nets for malaria protection, MDG 'villages', immunisations, school meals, and water purification devices. Investments of this kind can have a rapid pay-off for the MDGs, driving down key indicators for the goals, and helping to mobilise more donor funds. Most of them involve not systemic change but delivering individual health and education benefits.

Human rights standards also do not explicitly address inequality, concerning themselves primarily with establishing minimum standards and core protections. But human rights-based approaches to social policy do give a central role to probing root causes of poverty and ill-health, and identifying discriminatory practices and strengthening access to productive resources are, in principle, central. Several agencies adopting rights-based development approaches stress that human rights provide an improved framework for analysing causes of poverty (Sida, 2001). CARE has adopted methods that reflect the same view, including a 'rights-based monitoring tool' that relies on an analysis of discrimination to understand poor rural households' limited access to land, credit and agricultural inputs (Picard, 2004).

This difference appears at first to be one of strategy, but on closer examination, the MDG and human rights-based approaches differ more fundamentally. Most MDG strategies are neither societal nor systematic: the 'quick wins' strategy invests in measures that benefit individuals and households, for the most part, without creating social or institutional changes that can produce follow-on benefits for those not reached.

Embracing this strategy for a global anti-poverty initiative means that other possible strategies are de-emphasised. Structural factors accounting for poverty and wealth in poor countries – access to land, labour, wages and credit – are not touched on by the MDGs. The only attention given to discrimination is in the education goals, which aim to eliminate disparities between boys' and girls' enrolment levels. MDG proponents argue that because the goals are output measures, they do not exclude strategies that expand access to productive resources (Malloch-Brown, 2003), and critics of the MDGs have called for just this kind of broader effort to address the causes of poverty (Social Watch, 2005).

Human rights

Human rights and development practitioners have led a resurgence of interest in the economic and social human rights since the mid-1990s. Amnesty International and Human Rights Watch, for example, have begun to expand their focus from advocacy on civil and political rights to include economic, social and cultural rights (Nelson and Dorsey, 2007, 2008).

Among major donors, the Australian, British, Norwegian and Swedish aid agencies have adopted rights-based approaches. The UN agencies' experience is analysed in Darrow and Tomas (2005), while more recent studies document the bilateral and NGO experiences (for example, Plipat, 2006). Specialised ESC rights NGOs have also emerged, including the Centre on Housing Rights and Evictions (COHRE), the Food Information and Action Network (FIAN), the Centre for Economic and Social Rights (CESR), the International Women's Health Coalition and a global network of NGOs on ESC rights (ESCR-net.org).

Rights-based approaches are also a source of legitimacy for aid donors eager to occupy the 'high moral ground' associated with human rights (Uvin, 2002, pp 1-2). Uvin argues that 'incorporating human rights terminology into development discourse' is a rhetorical gesture that need not involve substantive changes in actual policies, projects or programmes. Aid agencies acknowledge these benefits; the UN Development Programme (UNDP, 2000), for example, claims that the union of human development and human rights 'can bring new energy and strength to the other' (2000, p 2) and that rights 'lend moral legitimacy' to human development (2001, p 3).

Human right to health

Human rights related to health and access to healthcare are spelled out in several of the major human rights agreements, most extensively in the International Convention on Economic, Social and Cultural Rights (ICESCR), whose Article 12 recognises every person's right to 'enjoyment of the highest attainable standard of physical and mental health'. Like other ESC rights, the right to health implies three kinds of obligations for states: to respect (avoid violating the right themselves), to protect (prevent others from violating the right) and to fulfil (by adopting appropriate policies, legal frameworks and other measures to work towards the full realisation of the right) (Committee on Economic, Social and Cultural Rights, 1966).

The practical difficulty of interpreting this standard led to a clarifying, authoritative General Comment 14 from the Committee on Economic, Social and Cultural Rights (2000). General Comment 14 gives a central place to accessibility and affordability of healthcare, the provision of safe water and basic sanitation and access to healthcare for marginalised groups. It identifies 'core obligations' that all states must meet immediately, including immunisation against basic infectious diseases, access to essential medicines and appropriate treatments for common diseases. The General Comment also specifies circumstances under which the right to health clearly is violated, including, among others, when governments enter into bilateral or multilateral agreements that compromise citizens' access to essential health services.

These clarifying efforts notwithstanding, the human right to health is often criticised as vague (Fidler, 1999), and arguably does not help in resolving some key policy dilemmas such as the tension between humanitarian imperatives and public health perspectives (Brauman, 2006). As with other social rights, some argue that the lack of a metric for making different allocation choices (as between funds to address malaria and HIV/AIDS) weakens the right to health as a development policy-making tool (Gauri, 2004).

But there is a growing record of jurisprudence on ESC rights, including those to housing and to health (COHRE, 2003). Moreover, there is a growing tendency, among national and transnational social movements, to embrace human rights standards as motivating principles and sources of political leverage, as well as for potential litigation. Political activism has rendered ESC rights debates more concrete and specific: human rights activists in the 1990s drew attention to the right to agrarian reform, as an implication of the right to food; and to the right of access to essential medicines, as a requirement of the right to health; and to the right to inheritance and secure property ownership for women, as a foundation for the right to housing.

Advocacy for the right of access to HIV/AIDS treatment has involved close cooperation with governments (Brazil, India and South Africa); strong North–South links between activist movements; and appeals to ESC rights standards as a counterweight to corporate power and to liberal trade rules (Nelson and

Dorsey, 2006). Friedman and Mottiar's (2005) study of mobilisation strategies of the Treatment Action Campaign (TAC) in South Africa demonstrates the impact of TAC's rights-based mobilisation strategy on government decisions to provide and finance treatment to HIV-positive citizens.

Whose goals and whose rights?

Goals and rights differ in theory, in their relations to individuals and governments, and these differences are fundamental to understanding the politics of ESC rights and of the MDGs. Human rights in some cases refer to groups (children, women and indigenous peoples) as the rights-holders, but the broad range of human rights contained in the Universal Declaration of Human Rights (UDHR), International Covenant on Economic, Social and Cultural Rights (ICESCR) and International Covenant on Civil and Political Rights (ICCPR) are rights of individuals. Each government that is party to a human rights agreement has duties defined by the treaty, to respect, protect and work towards fulfilling rights for all citizens. Governments, then, do not possess the rights in the sense that they possess rights and privileges under other treaties.

Goals, on the other hand, belong to states and the international organisations in which they are negotiated. They *refer* to the people who suffer the indignities of poverty, but those individuals are the objects of the goals, not their agents. The fact that governments affirm the goal of reducing by half the number of people living in extreme poverty does not give any particular destitute person a right or a claim on their government. Similarly, the fact that the goals aim for reductions by half (poverty), or by three quarters (maternal mortality), means that even in the event that one or more of the goals is accomplished in 2015, no individual is assured of any direct benefit. The MDGs are not individual citizens' goals in the same sense that the right to food or to information is their right.

Rights, unlike goals, inherently create duties that give them much of their political significance. The claim, for example, that each citizen of Niger has the right to adequate food, by virtue of their dignity as a human being, is a meaningful statement in the abstract: a dignified human life inherently involves freedom from hunger. But in political terms, the statement has meaning because it implies duties and obligations, and defining those duties is among the most difficult challenges for human rights. In this case, the duty to respond to acute malnutrition extends, under Article 2 of the ICESCR, to states and international agencies that are in a position to provide assistance, although the government continues to hold the principal responsibility to assure that resources are marshalled to protect its people (Frontline Defenders, 2005).

Mobilisation: MDGs, human rights and politics of global social change

A variety of social actors are important to achieving goals or fulfilling human rights. This section focuses on the ability of the MDGs and human rights standards and principles to mobilise one key set of actors, social movements and activist NGOs, particularly those based in the poor countries, and argues that the MDGs are much more relevant to development discourse in international circles than among Southern social movements and NGOs.

Advocates of the MDGs often refer to the goals' capacity to strengthen accountability. Fukuda-Parr (2004, p 397) of the UNDP argues that because the MDGs 'can be monitored', they create a 'framework for accountability', empowered by a 'systematic procedure for global monitoring and support' maintained by the UN. Indeed, the MDGs have spawned 'an industry of costing, planning and campaigning in the UN system, among donor governments, the IFIs [International Financial Institutions] and many CSOs [civil society organisations]' (Tomlinson, 2005). The 2006 report of the World Bank/International Monetary Fund's Development Committee goes further, calling the MDGs a route to 'mutual accountability' between donor and recipient countries (Development Committee, 2006).

But in practice, neither the MDGs nor ESC rights at present have an effective means of holding donors or governments accountable to their pledges or policies. Theoretically, ESC rights have the same legal authority as civil and political human rights, but suffer from very weak institutions crafted to monitor them within the UN Economic and Social Council (ECOSOC) (Felice, 1999).

Accountability 'outward' to a donor agency is rarely enough to promote the kind of social change envisioned in the MDGs. Mark Malloch-Brown (2002, p 6), UNDP Administrator, argues that while the MDGs' 'unique global authority' comes from their endorsement by 189 states, progress will come when 'everyone from a politician here in Berlin to a farmer in Bangladesh or a shop-keeper in Burkina Faso can understand and push for further action by their own governments…'. The campaign, Malloch-Brown argues, has to generate momentum, 'build[ing] on the success of global campaigns like the debt relief and land mines movements…' (2002, p 6).

In the absence of strong international authority and sanctions, Malloch-Brown is correct: if the MDGs are to stimulate change in policies, spending priorities and institutions in the poor countries, they must be able to mobilise local NGOs, community organisations, social movements and others in order to generate accountability within national political systems.

Poor country NGOs and social movements, and the MDGs

We have seen that senior UN officials emphasise the need for domestic social action in support of the MDGs. Eveline Herfkens (2006), Director of the UN's

Millennium Development Campaign, refers to the need for 'citizen pressure for change' to advance the goals; elsewhere, Herfkens (2005) calls on citizen groups to 'bring the MDGs to the streets'. Can the MDGs mobilise this kind of citizen action? One test of the relevance of the MDGs and human rights agreements to social movements and NGOs is the presence, or absence, of the MDGs from such organizations' public statements, documents and programmatic agendas. An inspection of publications, press releases and website documents provides some evidence of how relevant the MDGs are to social movements and development NGOs based in Southern societies.

(The investigation was based on the organisations' world wide web pages. Because some social movement organisations (Thailand's Assembly of the Poor, for example) do not have a web presence, this method likely biases the survey towards organisations *more* likely to be engaged with international processes. For each organisation, the website's internal search engine was first used to search for pages and documents with the keywords 'millennium' and 'millennium development goals'. Next, links to 'publications', 'campaigns', 'our work' and similar sections were followed. For websites without an internal search function, these links were used exclusively.) The organisations and their references to the MDGs and to human rights standards and principles are listed in Table 15.1.

Table 15.1: International and southern NGOs: links to human rights and MDGs

	Reference to human rights	Reference to MDGs	No reference
International NGOs	Doctors Without Borders International Women's Health Coalition	Oxfam CARE CRS World Vision Physicians for HR Action Aid Caritas Healthlink Worldwide Mercy Corps	Project Hope
Poor country-based NGOs and social movements	Greenbelt Movement (Kenya) SEWA (India) TAC (South Africa) People's Health Movement (Bangladesh) MST (Brazil)	AMREF (Kenya) Social Watch (Uruguay)	ARMS (India) CSI (India) BRAC (Bangladesh) PRRM (Philippines) CINI (India)

Eleven such movements and NGOs were examined to assess the political relevance of the MDGs to their work. Six of these are prominent, relatively large-scale NGOs and movements in the aid-recipient countries:

- Bangladesh Rural Action Committee (BRAC), Bangladesh;
- Greenbelt Movement, Kenya;
- Landless Workers' Movement (MST), Brazil;
- Philippine Rural Reconstruction Movement (PRRM);
- Self-Employed Women's Association (SEWA), India;
- Treatment Action Campaign (TAC), South Africa.

No reference to the MDGs was found on any of the NGOs' websites, even though each is working in areas directly referenced in the goals, and public advocacy is a central part of the organiaational mission for three (MST, SEWA and TAC).

Another five NGOs in the health sector, based in the global South, were surveyed with similar results. These organisations were:

- African Medical and Research Foundation (AMREF), based in Nairobi. AMREF documents make a single reference to the MDGs, but none makes reference to the MDGs as a source of leverage or motivation for mobilising political leverage or resources;
- Ashwinikumar Medical Relief Society, India, whose work focuses on tuberculosis;
- Centre for Science and Environment, a research and advocacy institute based in New Delhi, India;
- Child in Need Institute, India;
- People's Health Movement, based in Dhaka, Bangladesh.

References to human rights are more common, and recent literature on health policy advocacy campaigns by NGOs and social movements in Latin America (Shepherd, 2003) and South Africa (Friedman and Mottiar, 2004) conclude that social movements can rely heavily and successfully on human rights standards and the incorporation of those standards in national constitution and statute.

The MDGs have a much higher profile among international NGOs. Five such NGOs were examined:

- Action Aid;
- CARE-US;
- Caritas Internationalis;
- Catholic Relief Services (CRS) (US);
- Oxfam Great Britain.

Each of these makes reference prominently to the MDGs, as a policy framework for work in a sector or a specific project (CARE, CRS), as a framework for advocacy on debt, development aid and other issues (Action Aid), as the subject of an advocacy campaign (Oxfam Great Britain) or as the focus of a critical report (Caritas Internationalis).

The MDGs are also more prominent in the discourse of international health NGOs than of their Southern counterparts. Most make reference to the MDGs as well as to health-related rights (International Women's Health Coalition; Healthlink Worldwide). Some focus solely on human rights (Physicians for Human Rights, Doctors Without Borders); Project Hope, the US-based health services NGO, makes no explicit references to international or national policy.

The contrast between the two sets of NGOs – international and Northern versus national/regional, social movement-allied and Southern – suggests that while the UN and MDG organisers have had some success in reaching the interested and concerned population in the US and Europe, the MDGs have not become salient to major organisations and networks based in poor countries. This divide may be a matter of concern for observers of NGOs; for current purposes, it demonstrates the limitations of such goals as tools for internal political leverage over government policies.

Policy and politics: the divide between the MDGs and human rights

But if, despite the conceptual differences and contrasting constituencies, the MDGs and human rights approaches promoted a consistent global set of humane policy initiatives, the differences might be of purely theoretical interest.

Many human rights and development agencies take this position: Action Aid, Christian Aid, Misereor, Oxfam and others have aligned themselves with rights-based approaches and advocate the MDGs as a step towards the broader realisation of these rights. Shetty (2005), of the UN-sponsored Millennium Development Campaign, calls the MDGs the link between human rights and 'mainstream economic decision-making processes', such as those of the international financial institutions. Philip Alston (2005), advisor to the High Commissioner on Human Rights for the MDGs, also emphasises the potential for harmonisation and coordination, even as he stresses the MDGs' failures to emphasise their grounding in international human rights (Alston, 2005).

But there are stark disagreements and differences of emphasis among the organisations associated with health-related policy. The debates over water privatisation and the provision of anti-retrovirals illustrate these policy differences, and the strong tendency of those social actors affiliated with the MDG process and advocates of human rights approaches to square off on opposite sides of the issues.

Water

Advocates of the MDGs call for donors to step up their assistance for clean water supply and sanitation, and the major donors have complied, increasing investments in water in recent years. These new resources for potable water are being invested through country programmes that generally de-emphasise project funding, instead providing system-wide support to improve and expand water systems. Donor aid is overwhelmingly for the 'reform' of public utilities and to finance a shift to private sector provision, through contracts, franchises or outright ownership of formerly public water utilities. Human rights analysis and activism, on the other hand, has backed anti-privatisation campaigns.

Although water provision by private firms is a longstanding arrangement in a few countries (England, for one), the present rapid move towards private provision has its origins in the late 1980s. Donors have actively promoted the transition to private water provision. The World Bank's expanded investment in water under the MDG rubric has been largely to promote shifting water and sanitation utilities from government to private hands. At the international level, official policy favours market mechanisms and public–private partnerships to mobilise capital for water services. Months after General Comment 15 was released (Committee on Economic, Social and Cultural Rights, 2002), an international commission led by Michel Camdessus produced a global strategy for financing water that makes no mention of the human right to water, and gives priority to creating favourable conditions for investors as the means of meeting MDG water goals (Winpenny, 2005).

Water has inspired human rights claims directly and urgently. Price, affordability for low-income citizen-consumers and the corporate preference for prepayment arrangements have been the major factors triggering human rights-based resistance, as the experience in Ghana, India and South Africa illustrates. In a debate typical of others in Sub-Saharan Africa, the Coalition against Privatisation of Water in Ghana objected to the government's 'fast track' implementation of privatisation, and to the lack of transparency and perceived favouring of multinational corporations in negotiating to sell public water utilities (International Water Working Group, 2002). As elsewhere, they invoke international human rights (Ghana National Coalition against the Privatisation of Water, 2001).

In South Africa, national guarantees, contained in the 1994 Constitution that embraced many internationally recognised human rights standards, have allowed a powerful domestic challenge to privatisation efforts (SAMWU, 2000). The prepaid meters, which require advance payment for access to community water sources, have enabled advocates to make strong legal arguments against the privatisation contracts (Anti-Privatisation Forum, 2003; Conca, 2005).

In India, both human rights arguments and sentiment against transnational corporations figure prominently in legal and political challenges to the National Water Policy of 2002, which provided for private ownership and management of water systems (Pant, 2003); and in opposition to extensive corporate use of water resources, most notably in cases involving Coca Cola (Vidal, 2003).

A growing set of international NGO advocates are supporting these movements, particularly since the UN ESC Rights Committee's November 2002 clarification of the legal basis for a human right to water. Among these are the UK-based

NGO Water Aid (2003), the New York-based Center for Economic and Social Rights (CESR, 2004) and the International Water Working Group (2004). New reports and advocacy initiatives have been launched by the WHO (2002); Amnesty International (2003); Jubilee South (Laifungbam, 2003); the Centre on Housing Rights and Evictions (COHRE, 2004); the German NGOs Brot für die Welt and WEED (Hoering and Schneider, 2004); and WHO et al (2004).

This difference is not a matter of emphasis or strategy, it is a disagreement over the fundamental principles that guide the provision of water, as the rules and institutions that shape the power relations between international corporations and poor country governments are being reshaped in national and international settings.

Access to essential medicines

Advocates of MDGs and of human rights have agreed that malaria and HIV/AIDS are top health priorities. As with water and sanitation, the major donor countries and international organisations are encouraged to increase their investments in health and sanitation, and to contribute more generously to the UN Fund to Fight Tuberculosis, Malaria and AIDS. There is much debate over how adequately donors have followed through on commitments to the Fund (LaFraniere, 2004). But more fundamentally, activists have been at odds with the major donors and the trade rule-making process at the WTO.

While donors declare their support for making HIV treatment more widely available, some industrial country governments have continued to insist on patent protections for commercial drugs that drive up the cost of treatment (Cullet, 2003). AIDS activists appeared to win a partial victory in 2001, when the WTO Ministerial Meeting at Doha reaffirmed that governments' right to act in a public health emergency superseded intellectual property rights rules, and made a 15-year exception to key intellectual property rules.

But this ruling opened further debate over the mechanisms by which poor country governments can import generic drugs, with human rights activists calling for a low-cost and streamlined mechanism for trade in generics. The temporary mechanism adopted in December 2005 by the Ministerial Meeting in Hong Kong has been criticised as a 'burdensome and unworkable' solution whose case-by-case approach violates the spirit of the 2001 agreement giving priority to health rights ('Joint Statement by NGOs on TRIPS and Public Health', 2005).

Conclusion

The MDGs propose to mobilise donor and poor country governments, NGOs and social movements worldwide in support of a set of goals and initiatives to reduce rapidly some of the worst symptoms of extreme poverty. For the MDGs, the link to human rights, including economic and social rights such as the right to health, is an important source of legitimacy, and an important tie to social movements in the global South. This link is tenuous, I have argued, for two broad reasons.

First, despite the rhetoric of common global commitment to the MDGs, and MDG proponents' intention of winning broad support from NGOs and social movements, the social actors involved in the aid system have responded differently to the global development goals. It is no surprise that social movements on housing, HIV/AIDS, agrarian reform and water do not readily align themselves with the donor governments. Social movements' strength rests in their ability to press demands on their own governments and on international authorities, while donors prefer to set policy in terms that do not accede to rights-based demands.

But the divide between international development NGOs and the NGOs and social movements in the aid-recipient countries is more surprising. My preliminary review of poor country-based movements and NGOs suggests that the MDGs have little salience for them, and that many politically active NGOs and movements embrace ESC rights and use them to bolster the legitimacy and leverage of their demands.

There is an irony in this pattern of action. Human rights standards, which are binding on states' parties, might be expected to be the vehicle for concerted state action on development and health. They are instead the mobilising force for social movements and the networks that support them, while soft goals, which have no force of a treaty and have the ring of voluntary action, are the preferred vehicle for donor governments.

Second, this pattern of mobilisation also has implications for substantive policy issues, as the survey of HIV/AIDS and water privatisation debates shows. In the case of water, social movements of consumers, citizens and other activists have had some success in stalling, disrupting or scuttling contracts with transnational corporations to manage municipal water schemes in Africa, Asia and Latin America. But there is little evidence of similar effectiveness in using human rights or other arguments to win better service from existing or modified public utilities.

In the case of HIV/AIDS, activists and social movements have an abiding mistrust of the intentions of most of the major donor governments and agencies, grounded in their view that the US and the European Union will not voluntarily negotiate workable arrangements for a public health exception to patent protections of anti-retroviral drugs.

Goals and rights organise and motivate actors in the global aid and development system. The affinity of the major donor countries and institutions for soft goals, and the preference of the social movements for human rights-based demands, raises the stakes in the dialogue and interaction between the MDGs and human rights-based approaches. Understanding the nature and extent of the differences is a step towards more strategic and more fruitful interactions.

References

Alston, P. (2005)'Ships passing in the night: the current state of the human rights and development debate seen through the lens of the Millennium Development Goals', *Human Rights Quarterly* 27: 755-829.

Amnesty International (2003) 'World Water Forum Statement', 23 March.

Amnesty International USA (2006)'Health and human rights' (www.amnesty. usa.org/healthl/humanright.html).

Anti-Privatisation Forum (2003) 'The struggle against pre-paid water meters in Soweto', 10 September (www.labournet.net/world/0309/sawater1.html).

Bissio, R. (2003) 'Civil society and the MDGs', *UNDP Development Policy Journal* 3: 151-60 (www.undp.org/dpa/publications/DPJ3Final1.pdf).

Brauman, R. (2006) 'Questioning health and human rights', Carnegie Council on Ethics and International Affairs (www.cceia.org/printerfriendlymedia.php. prmID/643).

CESCR (Committee on Economic, Social and Cultural Rights) (1966) International Covenant on Economic, Social and Cultural Rights, adopted and opened for signature, ratification and accession by General Assembly Resolution 2200A (XXI) on 16 December 1966 (www.unhchr.ch/html/menu3/b/a_cescr. htm).

CESCR (2000) General Comment No 14, 'The right to the highest attainable standard of health', UN Doc E/C.12/2000/4.

CESCR (2002) General Comment No 15, 'The right to water', 27 November (www.waterobservatory.org/library/uploadedfiles/right _to_water_Articles_ 11_and_12_of_the_Inter.pdf).

COHRE (Centre on Housing Rights and Evictions) (2003) '50 leading cases on economic, social and cultural rights summaries', Geneva: COHRE (www. cohre.org/downloads/50leadingcases.pdf).

COHRE (2004) 'Legal resources for the right to water: National and International Standards', Source No 8, Geneva: COHRE (www.cohre.org/downloads/ water_res_8.pdf).

Conca, K. (2005) *Governing water: Contentious transnational politics and global institution building*, Cambridge, MA: MIT Press.

Cullet, P. (2003) 'Patents and medicines: the relationship between TRIPS and the human right to health', *International Affairs* 79(1): 139-60.

Darrow, M. and Tomas, A. (2005) 'Power, capture, and conflict: a call for human rights accountability in development cooperation', *Human Rights Quarterly* 27(2): 471-538.

Development Assistance Committee (2006) *Shaping the 21st century: The contribution of development cooperation*, Paris: OECD, May 1996 (www.oecd.org/ dataoecd/23/35/2508761.pdf).

Development Committee (2006) *Global Monitoring Report 2006: Strengthening mutual accountability – aid, trade and governance*, 23 April, Washington, DC: World Bank.

Felice, W.F. (1999) 'The viability of the UN approach to economic and social human rights in a globalized economy', *International Affairs* 3: 563-98.

Fidler, D.P. (1999) *International law and infectious diseases*, Oxford: Oxford University Press.

Friedman, S. and Mottiar, S. (2004) 'A rewarding engagement the treatment action campaign and the politics of HIV/AIDS', *Politics & Society* 33: 511-65.

Frontline Defenders (2005) *'National and international obligations', The right to development: obligations of states and the rights of minorities and indigenous peoples* (www.frontlinedefenders.org/manuals/91).

Fukuda-Parr, S. (2004) 'Millennium Development Goals: why they matter,' *Global Governance* 10: 395-402.

Gauri, V. (2004) 'Social rights and economics: claims to health care and education in developing countries,' *World Development* 32(3): 465-77.

Ghana National Coalition Against the Privatisation of Water (2001) Accra Declaration on the Right to Water (www.isodec.org.gh/Papers/accradeclaration. PDF).

Herfkens, E. (2005) 'Bring the MDGs on to the streets' (www.milleniumcampaign. org/site/pp.asp?c=grKVL2NLE&b=297468).

Herfkens, E. (2006) 'The Global Marshall Plan must generate citizen pressure for change', Guest Commentary on the Global Marshall Plan Initiative (www. millenniumcampaign.org).

Hoering, U. and Schneider, A.K. (2004) *King customer? The World Bank's 'new' water and its implementation in India and Sri Lanka*, Stuttgart: Brot für die Welt and World Economy, Ecology and Development.

Joint Statement by NGOs on TRIPS and Public Health, 3 December 2005 (www. cptech.org/ip/wto/p6/ngos12032005.html).

LaFraniere, S. (2004) 'UN fund for halting diseases faces money woes', *New York Times*, 17 April.

Laifungbam, D.R. (2003) 'The human right to water: necessity for action and discourse', Jubilee South (www.jubileesouth.org/news/EpZyVVlyFygMevRBey. shtml).

Malloch Brown, M. (2002) 'Meeting the Millennium challenge: A strategy for helping achieve the United Nations Millennium Development Goals' (www. inwent.org/ef-texte/mdg/brown.htm).

Malloch Brown, M. (2003) 'Millennium Development Goals, poverty reduction strategy papers and the new global development agenda, Address by the UNDP Administrator', New York, 14 February (www.undp.org/dpa/statements/ administ/2003/february/14feb03.html).

Meyer, J.W., Boli, J., Thomas, G.M. and Ramirez, F.O. (1997) 'World society and the nation-state', *American Journal of Sociology* 103(1): 144-82.

Nelson, P. and Dorsey, E. (2007) 'New rights advocacy in a global public domain', *European Journal of International Relations* 13(2): 187-216.

Nelson, P. and Dorsey, E. (2008) *New rights advocacy: Changing strategies of development and human rights NGOs*, Washington, DC: Georgetown University Press.

Picard, M. (2004) 'Measurement and methodological challenges to CARE International's rights-based programming' (www.enterprise-impact.org.uk/pdf/EINAug04.pdf).

Plipat, S. (2005) 'Developmentizing human rights: how development NGOs interpret and implement a human rights-based approach to development policy,' Unpublished doctoral dissertation, University of Pittsburgh.

SAMWU (South African Municipal Workers Union) and JRDSN (Joint Rural Development Services Network) (2000) Statement on the South African Water Services Act', Johannesburg, 21 August, on file with author.

Shepherd, B.L. (2003) 'NGO advocacy networks in Latin America: lessons from experience in promoting women's and reproductive rights', The North-South Agenda, Paper 61, February (www.ciaonet.org/wps/shb04/shb04.pdf).

Shetty, S. (2005) 'Making rights real: the challenge in meeting the MDGs', Public presentation, 24 March, London, Notes on file with the author.

Sida (2001) *Country strategy development: Guide for country analysis from a democratic governance and human rights perspective*, Stockholm: Sida.

Social Watch (2005) *A civil society benchmark for the 5-year review of the Millennium Declaration* (www.socialwatch.org/en/noticias/documentos/Benchmark_2005_eng.doc).

Tomlinson, B. (2005) 'The politics of the Millennium Development Goals' (www.realityofaid.org/themeshow.php?id=14).

UN Millennium Project (2005) *Investing in development: A practical plan to achieve the Millennium Development Goals* (www.unmillenniumproject.org/reports/index.htm).

UNDP (United Nations Development Programme) (2000) *Human Development Report 2000*, New York, NY: Oxford University Press.

Uvin, P. (2002) 'On high moral ground: the incorporation of human rights by the development enterprise', *Praxis* 17:1-11 (http://fletcher.tufts.edu/praxis/xvii/Uvin.pdf).

Vidal, J. (2003) 'Coke on trial as Indian villagers accuse plant of sucking them dry,' *The Guardian*, 19 November.

Water Aid (2003) 'Human rights approach to development' (www.righttowater.org.uk/code/HR_approach.asp).

WHO (2002) '25 questions & answers on health and human rights', Health and Human Rights Publication Series Issue no 1, July.

WHO, Centre on Housing Rights and Evictions and American Association for Advancement of Science (2004) *Manual on the right to water* (www.cohre.org/downloads/water_flyer.pdf).

Winpenny, J. (2005) 'Financing water for all: Report of the World Panel on Financing Water Infrastructure, chaired by Michel Camdessus, March 2003' (www.gwpforum.org/servlet/PSP).

SIXTEEN

What the public needs to know about social inequality and public health

Salvatore J. Babones

As fate would have it, the chain of events that eventually led to the publication of this book had its genesis in a chance encounter on the fringes of a homeland security meeting focused on responses to international terrorism. I had reported to the meeting that, despite reasonable-sounding suggestions to the contrary, social inequality did not really seem to be associated in any way with international terrorism. First of all, most international terrorism originates in middle-income countries, not poor countries. The people in those countries who become international terrorists are generally among the better off in their countries. On top of all this, international terrorist organisations are not generally (if at all) motivated by issues related in any way to social inequality. Despite the fact that I was invited to participate on the strength of my (presumably relevant) expertise in the area of social inequality, I found myself in the awkward position of having to argue that social inequality, in the end, just was not that important. The roots of international terrorism cannot be traced to social inequality.

A medical doctor who was also was also in attendance, a University of Pittsburgh psychiatrist named Kenneth Thompson, approached me after the meeting to ask me why, if social inequality was so unimportant, I spent so much time and energy studying it. The question was rhetorical: he had a ready answer. He told me that I should be studying social inequality because it was important for public health. He went on to argue, expansively but persuasively, that health (broadly construed to include happiness, contentedness, well-being and so on) was the only outcome that really mattered. To rail against inequality out of a preoccupation with social justice was immature: no one could really say what level of inequality was right or moral for a society. But we could establish – empirically – what level of inequality was healthy. The answer seems to be that the societies that today have the lowest levels of social inequality have the best health outcomes. Moreover, there does not seem to be any trade-off involved: such societies do not seem to be systematically poorer or worse off in any way. There is simply no excuse for high levels of social inequality.

That conversation inspired me to set out on a programme of learning, research and dissemination around the relationship between social inequality and public health, with the ultimate goal of influencing public policy in ways that would make the world a healthier place for all of us to live in. This effort has culminated in the present volume, which presents a wide range of perspectives (including my own) on the relationship between social inequality and public health, organised around the four broad causal pathways I found represented in the literature. The overall message of this book is very clear: social inequality has important implications for public health. Poor people have worse health than rich people; disadvantaged groups have worse health than advantaged groups; individual insecurity depresses individual health; harsh societies depress health for entire populations. Human beings are social animals – it should not be surprising that their social environments affect their health. Mice and monkeys respond biologically to social stimuli. So do we. The policy implications of this simple observation, however, can seem quite daunting.

The level of unhealthy individual health behaviours associated with or generated by social inequalities (Pathway 1) could be reduced through a very basic progressive policy agenda. We know that giving people greater hope for the future would encourage them to engage in better health-promoting behaviours (Chapter Two), but no one realistically expects sweeping New Deal-style public policies creating a right to work, advancement and personal fulfilment for all to be enacted on the basis of their potential public health benefits. We know that expanding public parkland and exercise facilities and incentivising healthy food stores to operate in low-income neighbourhoods might bring about a reduction in obesity (Chapter Three), with the added benefit that such policies have the potential to pay for themselves in lower government healthcare bills, but we know that few new parks have been built in our ageing cities since the 19th century. We know that implementing sustainable urban planning principles in the rapidly expanding population centres of the global South could prevent the proliferation of slums and instead channel population growth into healthy communities (Chapter Four), but we question the institutional capacity of governments in developing countries to implement such forward-thinking reforms.

The insidious effects of group advantage and disadvantage on health (Pathway 2) could be mitigated through targeted public policy interventions. We know that ensuring that public health interventions reach the entire population, rather than just advantaged early adopters, can prevent the expansion of health inequalities (Chapter Five), but we doubt the likelihood (or in some cases even the propriety) of government action to force new public health practices on potentially recalcitrant populations. We know that policies that promote equal opportunity for all can help break intergenerational cycles of poor maternal and child health (Chapter Six), but the progress of civil rights in the US at least has stalled and US communities are now more highly segregated by race than they were in the Jim Crow era. We know that non-governmental organisations are often the only bodies with the institutional capacity to serve the health needs of disadvantaged populations in the developing world (Chapter Seven), but aside from a few super-wealthy benefactors, most of us in the developed world are unwilling to part with even small sums of money to support their work.

The large but subtle influence of psychosocial factors (Pathway 3) could be channelled into improving, rather than depressing, individual health. We know that workplaces that give employees higher levels of personal autonomy and greater control over their own workflows are likely to have much healthier workforces (Chapter Eight), but technological trends are bringing about increasingly closely monitored, highly Taylorised working environments, even for high-income professionals. We know that social inequality can lead to the formation of fractured identities in society and thus exacerbate inter-group conflict (Chapter Nine), but the simple fact is that communal peace is a public good, and it is in no one's individual interest to redistribute their own wealth to bring about the greater good of societal harmony. We know that the collapse of communism created massive levels of social insecurity in Central and Eastern European economies, leading to a clearly measurable deterioration in health across the region (Chapter Ten), but the official Western policy at the time was precisely such 'shock therapy' to hasten those countries' transitions to capitalism.

The attributes that make entire societies healthy social environments in which to live (Pathway 4) are now well known and could be adopted by all societies. We know that extreme individualism and rampant consumerism poison both our social and our physical environments (Chapter Eleven), and outside a few self-interested pro-market think tanks hardly a voice can be heard today in defence of high-inequality social models, but few people seem interested in substituting the intangible reward of peace of mind for the material comfort of things. We know that population-wide government programmes like universal healthcare promote social solidarity and insulate against the worst effects of social inequality (Chapter Twelve), but recognise that politics in today's democracies is becoming ever more fragmented and polarised, making it increasingly difficult to legislate such sweeping policies. We know that societies characterised by high levels of income inequality suffer a depression in life expectancy of up to 10 years when compared to low-inequality societies (Chapter Thirteen), but the world's least healthy and most influential rich country is leading a coordinated worldwide programme of economic rationalisation that is quickly remaking the rest of the world in its own image.

I met Kenneth Thompson at a homeland security conference and set out on the course that led to the publication of this book because on September 11, 2001 nearly 3,000 Americans were murdered in a tragic series of coordinated terrorist attacks. The horror of those attacks should not be minimised. But it must be pointed out that in 2001 about 146 times as many Americans were killed by tobacco smoke as were killed by international terrorists. Similarly high ratios apply for Indonesia in 2002, Spain in 2004 and the UK in 2005. Taking a longer-term view, more than 3,000 times as many Americans have been killed by tobacco in the past 20 years as have been killed by international terrorists. Furthermore, while the so-called 'war on terror' has cost billions of dollars, rupiah, pounds, euros and so on (not to mention hundreds of thousands of human lives), simply outlawing tobacco would save the world billions of dollars, rupiah, pounds, euros and so on, far more than enough money to compensate all the vested interests who would lose out as a result of the ban. Outlawing tobacco is the ultimate public health no-brainer. And yet we have tobacco.

Like tobacco, social inequality is killing people in far larger numbers than international terrorism. While the deaths may be more difficult to identify than those due to smoking, they are widespread and well substantiated, as is evident from the science reported in this volume. Unlike tobacco, which is (sadly) persistently popular among large segments of the population, social inequality has few open advocates. No one argues passionately for their right to be excluded from public health advances, to live as a disadvantaged minority or to have their own healthcare underfunded. Few Americans turn down the free public health insurance they are offered on turning 65 years old; there is little reason to think that they would turn it down at younger ages, were it offered. Nor is it likely that such a system could be more expensive than the current US system, which spends more money to achieve worse health outcomes than any other peer country's health system. From a technocratic standpoint, the recommendations implicit in this book are, like outlawing tobacco, public health no-brainers.

What the public needs to know about social inequality and public health is that the obvious policy solutions, however unlikely they may seem on the surface, should actually be quite easy to implement in democratic societies. They are policies that would benefit an overwhelming majority of the electorate to the detriment of very small minorities that are very well positioned to bear the costs. Who does *not* believe in equal opportunity, public parks, good urban planning and the like? So if we all believe in these things, and we live in democratic polities, why do we not have these things? The trick, of course, is paying for the policies, but we know that low inequality is good for society, so taxing those who can afford to pay for such policies (and anyone with annual income in the six digits of dollars, euros or pounds can afford to pay) has the double benefit of both paying for the needed policies and reducing after-tax inequality. The essence of democracy is that the good of the many outweighs the good of the few, and it can hardly be construed as a trampling of minority rights to take a higher percentage (but not all) of individuals' income past their first few million dollars. Moreover, despite loud and repeated rhetorical claims to the contrary, there is no empirical econometric evidence linking high taxes on the wealthy to lower growth.

If the solutions are so obvious and so easy, why have they not been implemented? Sadly, the only real answer to this is that we do not really live in well-functioning democracies. For example, in 2000 the French electorate voted itself a 35-hour working week, down from a previous standard of 39 hours. This was the first major reduction in the standard working week in the developed world in just over a century. Such a reduction is certainly consistent with the policy lessons emerging from this book: shorter working hours mean liberation from workplace stress, more time to devote to exercise and healthy food preparation and greater opportunities for self-actualisation through leisure time. As it turned out, in the five years after this cut in working hours, economic growth in France was 42%

lower than it had been five years previously. Meanwhile, in the US, there was no change in the standard working week. Economic growth in the US was also 42% lower than it had been in the five years previously. Economic growth in Germany deteriorated by 68%. Clearly, the reduction in French growth was caused not by the reduction in working hours, but by a global economic slowdown. Nonetheless, French politicians used the reduction in growth as an excuse to abandon the 35-hour working week. Since then, growth has not rebounded – neither in France nor in the US. When politicians misconstrue data to persuade the electorate to accept policies that are not in the best interests of the electorate, democracy has failed.

At the core of the new public health is the realisation that public health is a public good. Laboratory bench epidemiology treats public health as a private good: each individual person exhibits behaviours and encounters environmental stimuli that help or harm their individual health. From a wider perspective, though, the social environment created by one individual affects other individuals. My willingness to pay taxes to support your cancer therapy encourages your willingness to vote for workplace regulations that ensure my annual vacation leave, and so on. Being surrounded by (physically, mentally and spiritually) healthy people makes me a healthier person. As with any other public good, the maintenance of public health requires constant vigilance, since every individual has an incentive to take private gains at the public expense. In democratic societies, this vigilance can and should be undertaken by governments, with the electorate watching the watchers. This should not be difficult: this is how good government is supposed to work. What the public needs to know about social inequality and public health is that it is possible to improve both, at the same time, at a reasonable (or non-existent) social cost. All it takes is the democratic will to do so.

Index